Gastrointestinal Tract Disease Syllabus

AMERICAN COLLEGE OF RADIOLOGY
PROFESSIONAL SELF-EVALUATION AND CONTINUING EDUCATION HOME STUDY PROGRAM

Elias G. Theros, M.D., *Editor*

COMMITTEE ON
PROFESSIONAL SELF-EVALUATION AND CONTINUING EDUCATION

Elias G. Theros, M.D., *Chairman*

Robert P. Barden, M.D.
Milton Elkin, M.D.
Harold G. Jacobson, M.D.
Theodore E. Keats, M.D.

Isadore Meschan, M.D.
Sidney W. Nelson, M.D.
E. James Potchen, M.D.
Philip Rubin, M.D.

SECTIONS

GASTROINTESTINAL DISEASE
Sidney W. Nelson, M.D.,
Chairman
Atis K. Freimanis, M.D.
Jerome Wiot, M.D.

CHEST DISEASE
Robert P. Barden, M.D.,
Chairman
Jack Edeiken, M.D.
William J. Tuddenham, M.D.

BONE DISEASE
Harold G. Jacobson, M.D.,
Chairman
Robert H. Freiberger, M.D.
Alex Norman, M.D.

GENITOURINARY DISEASE
Milton Elkin, M.D.,
Chairman
Joshua Becker, M.D.
Richard M. Friedenberg, M.D.
Erich K. Lang, M.D.

HEAD AND NECK DISEASE

Isadore Meschan, M.D.,
Chairman
James F. Martin, M.D.
Lee F. Rogers, M.D.

PEDIATRIC DISEASE
Theodore E. Keats, M.D.,
Chairman
Walter E. Berdon, M.D.
John A. Kirkpatrick, M.D.
Lionel W. Young, M.D.

NUCLEAR MEDICINE
E. James Potchen, M.D.,
Chairman
S. James Adelstein, M.D.
Frederick J. Bonte, M.D.
Russell C. Briggs, M.D.
Paul Hoffer, M.D.
C. Douglas Maynard, M.D.
Robert W. McConnell, M.D.
Kenneth R. McCormack, M.D.
Barbara J. McNeil, M.D.
Barry A. Siegel, M.D.

RADIATION THERAPY
Philip Rubin, M.D.,
Chairman
George Casserette, M.D.
David White, M.D.

CHEST DISEASE II
William J. Tuddenham, M.D.,
Chairman
Robert P. Barden, M.D.
Adele Friedman, M.D.
E. Robert Heitzman, M.D.

BONE DISEASE II
Robert H. Freiberger, M.D.,
Chairman
Jack Edeiken, M.D.
Harold G. Jacobson, M.D.
Alex Norman, M.D.

GENITOURINARY DISEASE II
Richard M. Friedenberg, M.D.,
Chairman
Joshua A. Becker, M.D.
Milton Elkin, M.D.
Erich K. Lang, M.D.

GASTROINTESTINAL DISEASE II
Jerome Wiot, M.D.,
Chairman
Atis K. Freimanis, M.D.
Roscoe E. Miller, M.D.
Sidney W. Nelson, M.D.

HEAD AND NECK DISEASE II
Lee F. Rogers, M.D.,
Chairman
James F. Martin, M.D.
Isadore Meschan, M.D.

PEDIATRIC DISEASE II
Walter E. Berdon, M.D.,
Chairman
Theodore E. Keats, M.D.
John A. Kirkpatrick, M.D.
Lionel W. Young, M.D.

PROFESSIONAL SELF-EVALUATION AND CONTINUING
EDUCATION PROGRAM

SET: 4
GASTROINTESTINAL TRACT
DISEASE
SYLLABUS

By

SIDNEY W. NELSON, M.D., Professor and Chairman, Department of Radiology, The
Ohio State University, Columbus, Ohio

ATIS K. FREIMANIS, M.D., Professor and Chairman, Department of Radiology, Medical College of Ohio at Toledo, Toledo, Ohio

JEROME WIOT, M.D., Professor and Chairman, Department of Radiology, University
of Cincinnati, Cincinnati, Ohio

Pediatric Consultant

THEODORE E. KEATS, M.D., Professor and Chairman, Department of Radiology, University of
Virginia, Charlottesville, Virginia

Questions prepared in cooperation with
The National Board of Medical Examiners

**Committee on Professional Self-evaluation and Continuing
Education, Commission on Diagnostic Radiology**

AMERICAN COLLEGE OF RADIOLOGY
Chicago, Illinois   1973

Composed and Printed at
    Waverly Press, Inc.

Author's Preface

"Examinations are formidable, even to the best prepared, for the greatest fool may ask more than the wisest man can answer."

Charles Caleb Colton (1780–1832)
Lacon, Or Many Things in Few Words
Vol. 1, #322

Keeping in mind Colton's admonition, the original Committee for Self evaluation and Continuing Medical Education set out to develop examination sets of 8- by 10-inch reproductions of roentgenograms and accompanying multiple-choice questions which would permit the examinee to indicate his diagnosis of each roentgenogram. These materials were to be sent to those radiologists interested in "self evaluation". Following the examination and return of the test materials, a mimeographed "answer syllabus" was to have been sent to each examinee, together with a set of 35-mm. black and white transparencies of the original test roentgenograms and additional colored transparencies of the pertinent pathological findings which might help the examinee better understand the roentgenologic findings shown on the reproductions of the test roentgenograms. However, it soon became obvious that this type of testing would not only be prohibitively expensive and inconvenient for the examinees, but would be lacking in many desirable features of a different type of examination, such as those which are being prepared by many specialty groups with the assistance of the National Board of Medical Examiners (NBME) including the written examinations of the American Board of Radiology. It was finally decided that a well-illustrated, multiple-choice type of examination would not only be far more economical than the original format, but would also provide a more objective and convenient way for each candidate to evaluate his knowledge of differential diagnosis.

We knew that a great amount of time and energy would have to be expended by the individuals responsible for developing the new format if the resulting examinations were to be practical, clinically oriented, fair, and yet challenging. Therefore, several members of our original Committee for Self-evaluation and Continuing Medical Education accepted the responsibilities as chairmen of the "subcommittees" established for the preparation of examinations in the diagnostic radiology of such major system areas as *chest, bone, genitourinary, gastrointestinal*, and *head and neck* radiology. It soon became apparent that it would be desirable to establish additional subcommittees in areas such as pediatric radiology and nuclear radiology. Although examinations will undoubtedly be prepared in additional subject areas in the future, the preparation of recurring examination "cycles" relating to the major body systems will probably require continuing efforts on the part of these hard-working subcommittees.

Each subcommittee learns a great deal from the examinations and syllabi published by the preceding subcommittees. We also learn much from the examinees themselves, many of whom we have a chance to talk to after they have taken the examinations. Although most of the criticisms we hear are constructive and helpful, we are anxious to listen to *all* opinions so that we may continuously improve our ability to provide the fairest and most meaningful examinations for practicing radiologists.

The goals of these examinations are twofold. First, they must *test knowledge*. However, it is equally important that they help *stimulate* the examinees to participate in a so-called "continuum" of learning. It is, of course, impossible to design the perfect examination, particularly for a field as broad as radiology, or, indeed, in the radiology of only *one* of the major body systems. Thus, the examination must be prepared in such a way as to "sample" an individual's knowledge of the area being tested. Although it would be desirable to have the examination consist primarily of many large *illustrations* of roentgenograms, this is prohibitively expensive and would also preclude the use of many additional test questions for each case which can test the radiologist's knowledge of roentgenologic differential diagnosis as well as his clinical knowledge. We believe that the format we are now using is a reasonable and practical method of testing, although it will be necessary to strive to develop ever better examinations.

Although all of the previous examinations have used the "A" type of multiple choice questions (the lead statement followed by five possible answers, one of which is the correct one), it was decided to add a little variety and interest to the gastrointestinal examination by including a certain number of "B" type ("association" or "matching") questions. Such questions are difficult to prepare, but if the comments and criticisms indicate that the examinees do better when confronted with a variety of question types, additional types of questions will probably be tried in future examinations.

With respect to the difficulty of the examination, it should be emphasized that this examination was not prepared with any preconceived idea of a planned difficulty level. Rather, the design is based upon the concept that it should be both *practical* and capable of *challenging* the *practicing* radiologist.

The examinee naturally wants to know how he "stacks up" with his colleagues and the demographic data uniquely permits him to compare himself with radiologists in all types of radiological practice. Since these examinations are available to any physician who wishes to take them, it is inevitable that many nonradiologists with a particular interest in the area of diagnostic radiology being tested will send for and take these examinations. However, since these examinations are prepared for radiologists, we believe they should score higher than nonradiologists; i.e., an examination for specialists in radiology should be able to discriminate between the radiologist for whom the examination was designed, as opposed to nonradiologists who have an interest in only one particular area. However, we also believe the examination should be designed so that practicing radiologists will be able to take a test which is not replete with questions dealing with esoteric conditions and useless information. Conversely, in order to be truly challenging and stimulating, the examination should contain a certain number of questions which require careful analytical thinking, and possibly a little struggling, in order to recall information which will result in the correct answers.

An answer syllabus can be prepared in many formats. The correct answer can be given to each question and a brief discussion can be given for each case used in the examination. However, as the chairman of the examination subcommittee on the gastrointestinal tract I have used my prerogative to prepare a syllabus which will hopefully clarify concepts which might otherwise require a great deal of searching, reading, and study on the part of the examinee. Possibly our subcommittee may have gone a little "overboard" on a few of our write-ups in the syllabus, and it would be useful for candidates to express their thoughts to the subcommittee in the interest of improving future answer syllabi. I also insisted that the illustrations of pathological material which are included in this syllabus would be *pertinent* to the understanding of roentgenological findings. Pathological material has not been included merely for the documentation of the correct diagnosis, but includes correlative types of pathological material. It was sometimes necessary to include microscopic sections (usually very low power) and some discussion of pathological physiology. Furthermore, a few diagrams and charts were used whenever it was thought they might help the examinee either reinforce what he already knew, or help to organize and clarify his thinking. If an examinee was unable to answer some questions in the examination he will be able to learn a good deal about those cases by studying the syllabus.

It is important to emphasize that the examination score for each examinee is known only by the examinee, since he receives the *one and only* copy of his answer sheet. The information previously extracted from his answer sheet regarding overall performance and the performance on each question is transformed into statistics which are punched on computer cards and *mixed, averaged,* and *collated* with the data from other examinees. This makes possible the preparation and publication of the final demographic data which enables the examinee to compare his own performance with that of other radiologists (or nonradiologists) in different types of radiological practices and settings. Thus, the threat of misuse of the individual examinee's examination results does not exist because no record is kept of the examinee and his score is not identified. This method of providing anonymity justifies the time-consuming labors of the testing subcommittees and the growing enthusiasm of practicing radiologists, since the original purpose of these self-evaluation examinations is being fulfilled.

The examination subcommittees will continue to make diligent efforts to prepare increasingly effective examinations in the future. In fact, as this page is being read, the hard work is already underway for the preparation of the *next* examination and syllabus on gastrointestinal tract diseases! The membership of the examination subcommittees will change, and with respect to the appointment of new members, an effort will be made to represent a different geographic area of the country. We also hope to include practicing radiologists on the subcommittees. However, the busy radiologists on these subcommittees must do much of this work on their own time. Thus, it will immediately become obvious to a new subcommittee member that the members of present and previous subcommittees are, indeed, highly motivated radiologists who are trying to do their best to help perpetuate the specialty of radiology for what it is; i.e., one of the most useful and fascinating branches of medicine.

The following textbooks were particularly helpful in the preparation of the gastrointestinal tract examination and syllabus, and they are recommended sources of information for radiologists who wish to further clarify topics described in the syllabus, and who wish to continue their acquisition of knowledge about gastrointestinal tract radiology:

Abrams H: *Angiography*, 2nd ed. Little, Brown & Co, Boston, 1971

Ariel IM, Kazarian KK: *Diagnosis and Treatment of Abdominal Abscesses.* Williams & Wilkins Co, Baltimore, 1971

Boley SJ (editor): *Vascular Disorders of the Intestine.* Appleton-Century-Crofts, New York, 1971

Bockus HL: *Gastro-enterology, Vols I, II, and III*, 2nd ed. WB Saunders Co, Philadelphia, 1964

Buckstein J: *The Digestive Tract in Roentgenology, Vols I and II*, 2nd ed. JB Lippincott Co, Philadelphia, 1953

Caffey J: *Pediatric X-Ray Diagnosis, Vols I and II*, 6th ed., Year Book Medical Publishers, Chicago, 1972

DiDio LJ, Anderson MC: *The Sphincters of the Digestive System.* Williams & Wilkins Co, Baltimore, 1968

Epstein BS: *Clinical Radiology of Acute Abdominal Disorders.* Lea & Febiger, Philadelphia, 1958

Frimann-Dahl J: *Roentgen Examinations in Acute Abdominal Diseases*, 2nd ed. Charles C Thomas, Springfield, Illinois, 1960

Golden R, Cimmino C, Collins LC, Dreyfuss JR, Janower ML: *The Digestive Tract.* In LL Robbins (ed): *Golden's Diagnostic Radiology, Section 5.* Williams & Wilkins Co, Baltimore, 1969

Gross RE: *The Surgery of Infancy and Childhood.* WB Saunders Co, Philadelphia, 1953

Lasser EC: *Dynamic Factors in Roentgen Diagnosis.* Williams & Wilkins Co, Baltimore, 1967

Margulis AR, Burhenne HJ: *Alimentary Tract Roentgenology, Vols II and II.* The CV Mosby Co, St Louis, 1967

Marshak RH, Lindner AE: *Radiology of the Small Intestine.* WB Saunders Co, Philadelphia, 1970

Meschan I: *Roentgen Signs in Clinical Practice.* WB Saunders Co, Philadelphia, 1966

Michels NA: *Blood Supply and Anatomy of the Upper Abdominal Organs.* JB Lippincott Co, Philadelphia, 1955

Paul LW, Juhl JH: *Essentials of Roentgen Interpretation*, 3rd ed. Harper & Row Publishers, New York, 1972

Schinz HR, Baensch WE, Friedl E, Uehlinger E: *Roentgen Diagnostics, Vol IV.* Grune & Stratton, New York, 1954

Shanks SC, Kerley P: *A Textbook of X-Ray Diagnosis, Vol on Abdomen*, 4th ed. WB Saunders Co, Philadelphia, 1968

Shehadi WH: *Clinical Radiology of the Biliary Tract.* McGraw-Hill Book Co, New York, 1963

Templeton FE: *X-Ray Examination of the Stomach*, revised ed. University of Chicago Press, Chicago, 1964

Wise RE: *Intravenous Cholangiography.* Charles C Thomas, Springfield, Illinois, 1962

The preparation of an examination and syllabus is not possible without the moral support and active help of many people. Dr. Milton Elkin, the Chairman of the Commission on Radiological Diagnosis of the American College of Radiology, gave much support to the Committee on Self-evaluation and Continuing Education and was always ready to advise, encourage, and help. His support and friendship are greatly appreciated.

Dr. Elias G. Theros, the chairman of our original committee from the outset, has been diligent and highly effective in organizing and directing the activities of the committee, and the subsequently formed subcommittees, toward the goal of helping practicing radiologists learn to evaluate themselves. His patience, irrepressible energy, and administrative skills are invaluable in such an important and vast undertaking.

Dr. Theodore E. Keats submitted pediatric cases and was the pediatric consultant for the committee. Although future examinations in pediatric radiology will preclude the use of pediatric cases in the other system areas, Dr. Keats' counsel has been greatly appreciated with respect to the pediatric cases included in the examinations and syllabi.

Mr. Earle V. Hart, of the American College of Radiology, has been a joy to work with. His good humor and deep understanding of the many other demands which occasionally interfered with desired progress toward the completion of the examination and syllabus are greatly appreciated. Never demanding, always helpful, and uniquely knowledgeable in the field of medical writing and publications, his contributions to the success of this important ACR-sponsored venture are of inestimable value.

I am particularly indebted to Martha Hughes for her work on many of the illustrations and her typing of much of the manuscript. Her help and suggestions were invaluable.

My secretary, Mrs. Nadine Heinlen, somehow was able to keep me "on schedule" during the past 2 years during which my commitments and responsibilities were, at times, almost intimidating. Nevertheless, her frequent reminders, her arrangements of meetings, her good judgment in handling calls from members of our subcommittee and the other individuals mentioned above, were handled with patience and tact and are much appreciated.

I am grateful for the skillful help of Mr. William Ollila, medical artist par excellense, who somehow was able to convert my clumsy sketches into illustrations which clearly convey the intended meaning.

Mr. Robert Jones showed infinite patience in making the photographic prints, and the high quality of the illustrations is a tribute to his photographic and dark room skills.

The radiological-pathological correlations were made possible by the conscientious assistance of my erstwhile peripatetic pathologist colleagues, Drs. William Holaday and Dieter Assor. The sincere interests shown by these two friends, and the delight they seemed to take in helping provide me with correlative pathological materials, are indicative of the often unacknowledged talents which contribute to the preparation of such an educational venture. In fact, our collaboration in the preparation of this syllabus on gastrointestinal tract disease has recently resulted in similar joint efforts to present some innovative teaching exercises to our medical students.

Drs. Atis Freimanis and Jerry Wiot, as the other members of the subcommittee, did much to make this venture successful. Their willingness to make trips to Columbus, their good humor in responding to my requests as we pressed toward certain deadlines, and their conscientious preparation of their material were greatly appreciated. Dr. Freimanis' secretary, Mrs. Sue Hughes, and Dr. Wiot's secretary, Mrs. Mary Ellen Meyer, also receive much credit for helping these busy people accomplish their goals.

I also thank Dr. William Howard, chief of the radiology department at the Columbus Childrens Hospital, for allowing us to use cases from his files.

Dr. Thomas Lloyd, chief radiology resident at the Ohio State University Hospitals, was helpful in obtaining certain references. He and other radiology residents and staff members too numerous to mention by name were all helpful in bringing to my attention cases which they thought might be useful.

Drs. Robert Zollinger and Luther Keith, my surgical colleagues, and Dr. Floyd Beman, my longtime gastroenterologist friend, had patients who were the subjects of many of these roentgenograms and correlative pathological materials used in this syllabus. To them particularly I give my heartfelt thanks for both their direct and indirect help.

Finally, those of us in the American College of Radiology who have been entrusted with the responsibility for helping to advance the cause of radiological education are thankful for the confidence shown in us, and we will continue to try to develop ever better methods of self evaluation for practicing radiologists.

Sidney W. Nelson, M.D.

Editor's Preface

Doctor Sidney Nelson, in his preface, has given such a thorough summary of the backgrounds, progress, and plans for the Self-Evaluation and Continuing Education program that your Editor feels he can add little and would like briefly to emphasize certain points.

First of all, I would like to thank Doctor Nelson for his consummate effort. He and his co-authors, Doctors Atis Freimanis and Jerome Wiot, have succeeded in developing the gastrointestinal package into a splendid model that we would all do well to emulate. The craftsmanship with which they have interwoven the syllabus around the examination material and the illustrations is a joy to behold. We are in the debt of Doctor Nelson and his co-workers. I am acutely aware of the long and painstaking labor that went into this. As a result, the reader is in for a very rewarding experience as he peruses the pages of this syllabus.

As has been emphasized previously, the College realizes that home-study programs conducted by mail are necessarily limited in scope and cannot possibly be but a small part of the evaluation of the effectiveness of a radiologist in his day-by-day practice. There are a host of activities in a busy day in the radiologist's office which cannot be measured by home-study packages. At best, the present materials measure principally the radiological lore and background of information needed for interpretation of radiological findings. Self-evaluation in other factors that determine competence as a radiologist requires different programs. Such programs, in fact, are now being developed by the College in a realistic attempt to provide full opportunities for self-evaluation and continuing education in all aspects of radiologic practice. For the moment, then, the reader should consider these present home-study packages as a means of exploring his fund of knowledge and his capacity for analyzing and synthesizing information to make radiologic diagnoses that are fairly challenging.

The choices of material for testing hopefully will provoke the reader into thinking closely about alternatives and compel his careful attention to the discussions in the syllabus. By so doing, we feel that the radiologist will get more thoroughly involved and derive the maximum benefit from the experience. Selected readings are provided which he may consult for further elucidation once he has developed momentum in his desire to learn from being piqued by the difficulty or even controversial nature of a question. When the participant realizes that the purpose of these packages is not really to test *per se* but to use the test as a primer to get him "hooked", and thus drive him to investigate (through the syllabus and its reading suggestions) the plausibility of his preferred answers and decisions, then he will finally appreciate that the main thrust of this program is continuing education through inculcating the desire to continue learning.

This syllabus, then, is intended to be the authors' discussion with the reader about the significance and the differential possibilities of the radiology in the test cases. Written tests and home-study packages are an excellent means to help the radiologist acquire the background he needs for interpretation. They go beyond textbooks and journal articles because they provide an interface with the author that more effectively conveys the experience of the author to the enrollee. They weigh a problem together, and the enrollee witnesses its solution by the author. He is also led to specific and selected reading references which bear on the peculiarity of the differential diagnostic problem in hand. Such a tack has been taken in texts and articles but examples of it are precious few.

The Editor again wishes to thank the American College of Radiology Staff which continue their meticulous attention to details for excellence. Thanks are particularly due Mr. Earle V. Hart, Jr., and Mr. William K. Melton without whose remarkable dedication and patience, the program would be impossible to launch and sustain. Special thanks are also due Doctor Milton Elkin in his capacity as Chairman of the mother Commission on Diagnostic Radiology, and as a member of the original Committee on Self-Evaluation and Continuing Education. His support and contributions have been varied and continuous.

Finally, all of the members of the committee join me in thanking all radiologists for their record-breaking response to this program. To date we have recorded over 6,500 subscriptions for Set I on Chest, 8,500 for Set II on Bone, and 5,500 for Set III on the Genitourinary Tract. The present volume on the Gastrointestinal Tract has already passed 5,000, and continues to grow apace. This makes our long hours of preparation seem worthwhile indeed, and at the same time it heightens our sense of responsibility. We fondly hope that as the program develops we can look forward to more of your critiques which will help shape future packages. We thus hope to sharpen the quality of both product and author and continue to build into radiology a new resource for continuing education.

Elias G. Theros, M.D.
Editor and Chairman

Gastrointestinal Tract Disease Syllabus

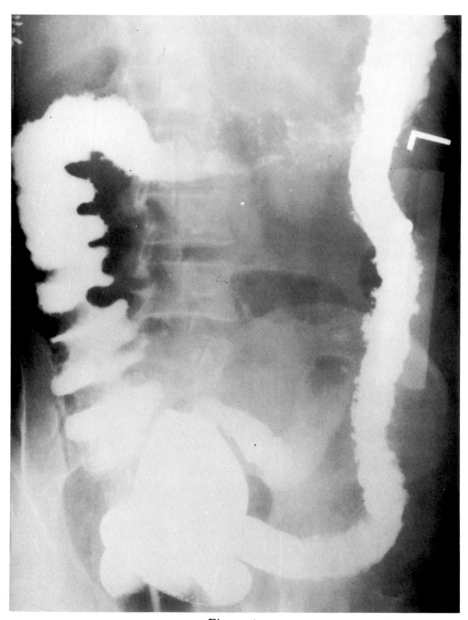

Figure 1

Figures 1 and 2. This 55-year-old man has diarrhea. Figure 1 is a left posterior oblique roentgenogram of the colon, and Figure 2 is an anteroposterior roentgenogram of the left side of the colon.

Questions 1 through 6

1. Which one of the following is the *MOST* likely diagnosis?

    (A)   Granulomatous colitis
    (B)   Acute vascular occlusion
    (C)   Ulcerative colitis
    (D)   Amebic colitis
    (E)   Cathartic colon

2. The *MOST* common complication of granulomatous colitis is

    (A)   hemorrhage
    (B)   fistula
    (C)   obstruction
    (D)   carcinoma
    (E)   perforation

3. Which one of the following roentgenographic signs is *MOST* characteristic of acute vascular occlusion of the colon?

    (A)   "Collar button" ulcers
    (B)   "Thumbprinting"
    (C)   "String" sign
    (D)   "Stack of coins"
    (E)   "Coil spring"

4. Which one of the following findings is *LEAST* characteristic of ulcerative colitis?

    (A)   Involvement of the rectum
    (B)   Circumferential involvement
    (C)   "Skip" areas
    (D)   Diffuse dilatation
    (E)   Perforation

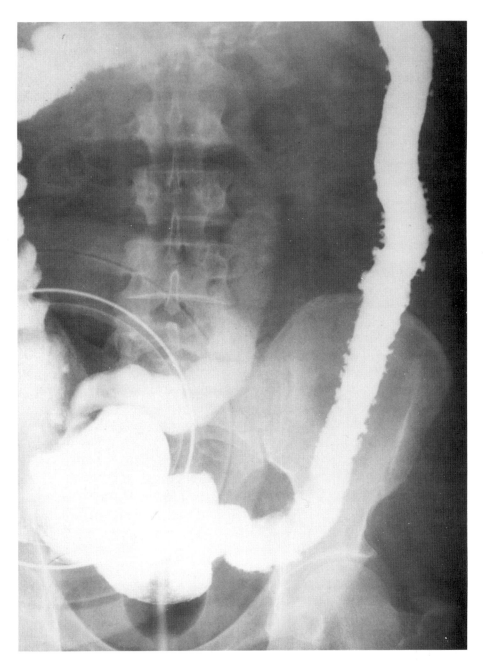

Figure 2

5. The *LEAST* frequent single site of extracolonic involvement in amebiasis is the

   (A) lung
   (B) brain
   (C) liver
   (D) peritoneum
   (E) small bowel

6. Which one of the following roentgenographic findings is *LEAST* characteristic of a cathartic colon?

   (A) Smooth contours
   (B) Effaced mucosa
   (C) Inconstant areas of narrowing
   (D) Poor evacuation of barium
   (E) Ulceration

Discussion

QUESTION 1

   These illustrations show evidence of ulcers distributed throughout almost the entire colon. The ulcers are largest on the left side where several are undermined (*arrows* in Figure 2B), whereas on the right side the ulcers are smaller and somewhat spiculated in appearance (*arrows* in Figure 2A). The undermining of the ulcers often produces the so-called "collar button" appearance (*white arrows* in Figure 2B, and in Figure 2C which is an enlargement of one of the undermined ulcers). Note that the disease involves the *entire circumference* of the colon as manifested by the fact that multiple *marginal* ulcers are seen in *all* projections. The circumferential distribution of the disease and the continuous involvement of one segment of the colon (in this case from the cecum to the sigmoid) are characteristic of acute ulcerative colitis, which is the diagnosis in this case. Therefore, **the correct answer to question 1 is (C).** It is also typical for this disease to be associated with a rather patulous ileocecal valve and a somewhat dilated terminal ileum (the so-called "backwash ileitis") which is well shown in Figure 2B ("*T.I.*").

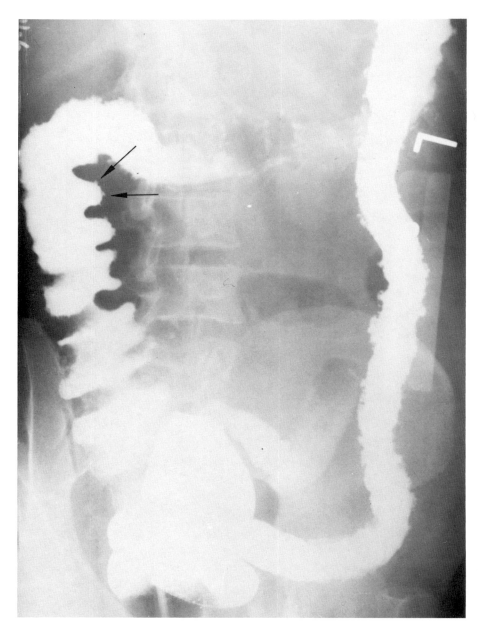

Figure 2A

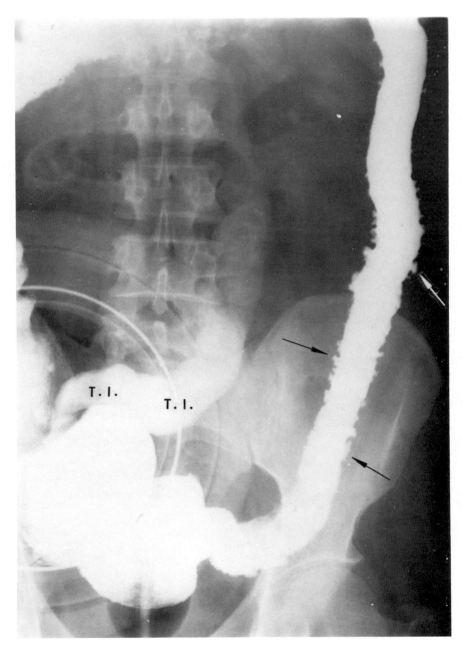

Figure 2B

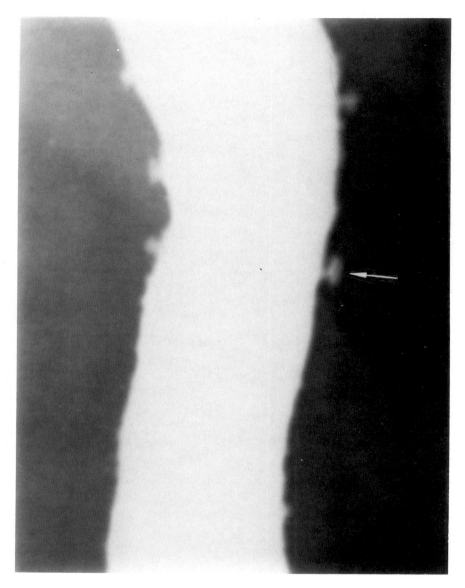

Figure 2C

It is not common for granulomatous colitis to involve such a long segment of colon in continuity. Granulomatous colitis usually involves more limited portions of the colon, often only on the right side. Furthermore, there is often more than one area of involvement with *intervening normal areas*. Such separate diseased areas are called "skip lesions". In contrast to the circumferential changes seen in ulcerative colitis, the involvement in granulomatous colitis is often *eccentric*; i.e., it involves only one portion of the

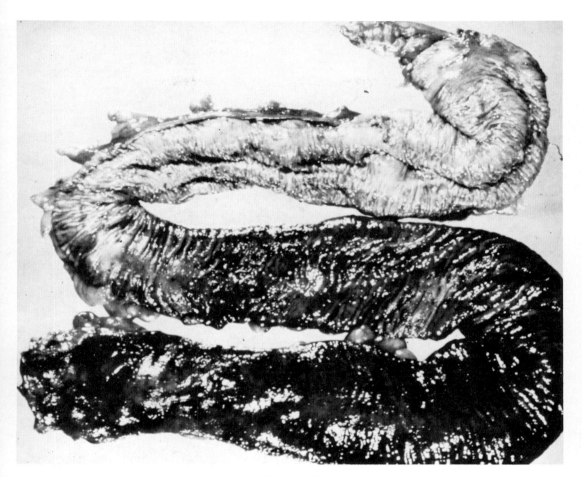

Figure 2D

circumference of the colon (see Figures 36A and B, p. 178). The tiny ulcers which produce the "spiculated" appearance (Figure 2A, *arrows*) and the "collar button" appearance (*white arrows* in Figures 2B and C) due to the undermining of the mucosa are probably more common in ulcerative than in granulomatous colitis, in which disease the ulcers are often in the form of slowly developing fissures or ulcers which are typically oriented longitudinally or transversely (see Figures 36A, B, and C, pp. 178–179). Furthermore, in granulomatous colitis the terminal ileum is often involved, in which case there will be an irregular, narrowed lumen owing to mucosal destruction and granulomatous thickening of the wall, in contrast to the dilated terminal ileum with a smooth or slightly granular mucosal surface which is so characteristic of ulcerative colitis. None of the typical changes of granulomatous colitis is seen in the case illustrated here.

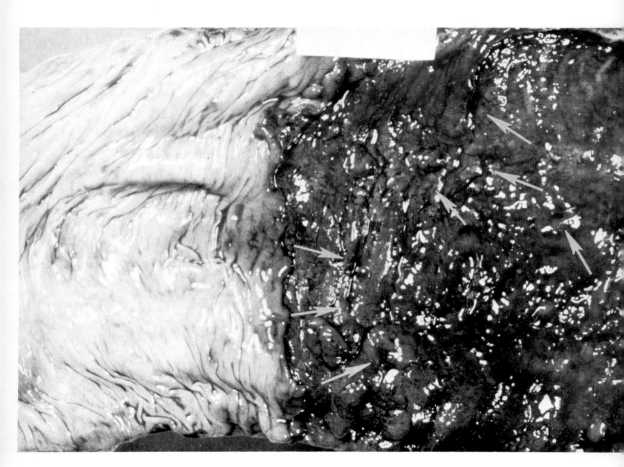

Figure 2E

The generalized involvement of almost the entire colon virtually precludes an acute vascular occlusion, because the extensive changes seen here would not be possible unless both the superior and inferior mesenteric arteries were involved. Such extensive ischemic disease would almost certainly be characterized by a fulminating clinical picture, in contrast to the primary complaint of diarrhea in the patient whose barium enema is illustrated here. Furthermore, acute vascular occlusion is usually characterized by submucosal hemorrhage with resultant "thumbprinting" and "transverse ridging" (see *arrows*, Figures 28A and B, pp. 142 and 143), neither of which is seen here. The findings of vascular occlusion are usually localized to shorter segments of either the right or left side of the colon.

It is true that amebic colitis can produce undermined ulcers, and it is sometimes impossible to differentiate this disease from acute ulcerative colitis. In amebiasis there is a predilection for the cecal and rectosigmoid

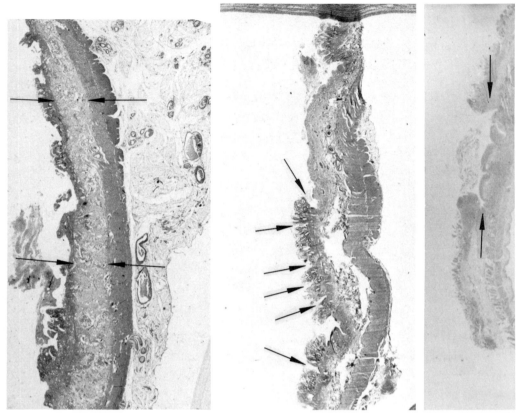

| Figure 2F | Figure 2G | Figure 2H |

areas, but it is unusual for the disease to involve the entire colon as seen in this case. The ileum is rarely involved. Most patients with amebiasis are relatively asymptomatic, and only a small percentage of patients will develop the clinical and roentgen picture of acute ulcerative colitis. Thus, on a stastistical basis alone, the roentgen appearance in this case suggests ulcerative colitis as a far *more likely* possibility than the rare case in which amebiasis will simulate acute ulcerative colitis.

Cathartic colon is not associated with ulcers. It may affect virtually the entire colon, but involvement distal to the splenic flexure is unusual. It is characterized by a smooth mucosa, in contrast to the irregular ulcerated mucosa seen in this case. In cathartic colon there are smoothly tapered narrow areas due to the sustained tonus of the circular muscle as a result of the chronic use of laxatives. These contractions resemble strictures, but are *not constant* and will slowly *change* in caliber. The areas of colon between these contracted segments may actually appear *wider* than normal, and there is a noticeable absence of haustra, all of which changes are probably due to the abnormal sustained tonus of the circular and longitudinal muscles caused by the particular laxatives used. None of these changes is seen in this case.

QUESTION 2

The correct answer to question 2 is (B) because the most common complication of granulomatous colitis is fistula formation. The fistulae may occur between the colon and adjacent small bowel, or as rectal fistulae which communicate with the skin in the anal region or with the vagina in females. There may also be intramural fistulae in the thickened wall of the colon. Although a fistula in the anal region may, on rare occasion, be seen in a patient with ulcerative colitis, it is far less common than the fistulous complications of granulomatous colitis.

Blood in the stools is far more frequent in ulcerative colitis than in granulomatous colitis. Conversely, obstruction, usually partial, occurs more frequently with granulomatous colitis, although it is a less common complication than fistula.

Although carcinoma of the colon has been reported occasionally in patients with granulomatous colitis, it is a much *more common* late complication of ulcerative colitis in which disease the incidence of carcinoma is reportedly twenty-five times greater than in patients who do not have ulcerative colitis.

Perforation is also more common in ulcerative colitis, particularly if the patient develops toxic megacolon, a condition in which the wall of the colon is thin and friable, and, therefore, easily ruptured during distention. Barium enema studies are contraindicated when toxic megacolon occurs because of the additional distention and danger of perforation caused by this study.

QUESTION 3

It is generally agreed that the most suggestive roentgenographic sign of acute vascular occlusion is "thumbprinting." Therefore, **the correct answer to question 3 is (B).** "Collar button" ulcers are not characteristic of acute vascular occlusion.

The "string sign" is seen in the chronic "stenotic" stage of granulomatous disease of the small intestine and is due to the marked narrowing of the lumen and thickening of the wall. The "stack of coins" appearance is seen in acute infarction, but usually occurs later than the "thumbprinting". The "coil spring" appearance is seen in patients with intussusception, and is not seen in patients with acute vascular occlusion.

QUESTION 4

The correct answer to question 4 is (C), because of the possible answers listed, "*'skip' areas*" is the *least* characteristic of ulcerative colitis. In fact, it is virtually unheard of to have different areas of ulcerative colitis separated by normal mucosa. All of the other possible answers in question 4 are findings commonly seen in ulcerative colitis.

QUESTION 5

Although the small intestine is almost never involved in amebiasis, amebic abscesses may occur in the liver, brain, lung, and peritoneum. Therefore, **the correct answer to question 5 is (E).**

QUESTION 6

The correct answer to question 6 is (E). All of the other listed possible answers are characteristic roentgen findings of cathartic colon.

DISCUSSION

The circumferential nature of ulcerative colitis and the tendency for the involved area to be one *continuous* segment is well demonstrated in the picture of the gross specimen of a patient with acute ulcerative colitis (Figure 2D). The involved segment (*dark area* in Figure 2D) is red, acutely inflamed, and ulcerated. Note that the disease involves the *entire width* of the rectum (*bottom left* in Figure 2D), sigmoid, and descending colon which are also involved in *continuity*. The wall of the colon is not appreciably thickened, but is rather soft and friable because the disease is primarily limited to the mucosa and submucosa.

Figure 2E is a close-up view of the transition between the normal (*light*) and abnormal (*dark*) areas of the colon. The highlights in the photo make it difficult to see the numerous undermined ulcers (*arrows*) in the markedly inflamed mucosa.

Figures 2F, G, and H show the characteristic microscopic manifestations of acute ulcerative colitis. The mucosal surface (at the reader's left in all sections) is shaggy and irregular due to the multiple ulcers, many of which extend into the somewhat edematous submucosa (the relatively *light-colored layer between arrows* in Figure 2F). The muscularis which comprises the thickness of approximately one-third of the bowel wall (*dark layer on right side* of Figure 2F) is not involved. The "spiculated" appearance (*arrows* in Figure 2A) is due to the small closely grouped ulcers (*horizontal arrows* in Figure 2G) which are not undermined, in contrast to the "collar button" shape of the ulcers associated with mucosal undermining (*top arrow* Figure 2G, and *vertical arrows* in Figure 2H).

Admittedly, about one-fourth of the patients with ulcerative colitis and granulomatous colitis will have some overlapping of the clinical, radiological,

Table 1
Differential Diagnostic Features of Ulcerative and Granulomatous Colitis

Differential Diagnostic Features	Ulcerative Colitis	Granulomatous Colitis
Circumferential *versus* eccentric involvement	Circumferential	Asymmetrical (eccentric)
Anatomic distribution of areas of involvement	May be *regional* or *segmental;* often limited to left side of colon. Entire colon often affected.	Entire colon usually not involved. One or more limited areas of involvement are common. May be limited entirely to right side of colon.
Ulcers	Characteristically many "collar button" ulcers with considerable undermining. Often develop pseudopolyps (smaller than "cobblestones").	May have "collar button" ulcers. Longitudinal and transverse ulcers ("fissuring") are more characteristic of granulomatous colitis. Often develop "cobblestoning".
Rectal involvement	Common	Uncommon
Skip areas	*Uncommon.* Usually one continuous area of involvement.	*Common.* Separate areas of involvement with normal areas between.
Terminal ileum involvement	When "backwash" ileitis is present, valve is wide open and terminal ielum is often dilated. No organic narrowing.	When right side of colon is involved, ileum is almost always involved. Usually ileocecal valve and terminal ileum are *narrowed* due to granulomatous thickening of wall and encroachment on the lumen.
Pseudo "tics"	Do not occur because of symmetrical involvement of *entire circumference* of colon.	Common because of eccentric involvement. Associated spasm and fibrosis cause shortening of diseased side. Folding (or "buckling") of opposite normal wall causes appearance of "pseudodiverticula".
Pathology	Granular, friable ulcerated mucosa. Vascularity often intense (see *dark areas* in Figures 2D and E).	Chronic inflammation. Noncaseating granuloma is characteristic. Much edema and fibrosis; many Langhans cells. Earliest changes are mucosal and submucosal edema and variable sized ulcers or fissures. Mucosa may appear relatively normal between ulcers or fissures (see normal mucosa between large ulcers and fissures in Figures 36C).

Table 1—*Continued*

Differential Diagnostic Features	Ulcerative Colitis	Granulomatous Colitis
Degree of involvement of colon wall	Usually limited to mucosa and submucosa. *Shortening* of colon often due to spasm of longitudinal muscle. *Diminished* caliber of colon due to spasm of circular muscle.	Granulomatous changes. All three layers of wall involved, especially submucosa. Wall thick and rigid. Lumen may be markedly narrowed.
Relationship to regional enteritis	None	Inflammatory colon disease in the presence of regional ileitis is *virtually always* granulomatous.
Response to medical management	Remissions may be complete.	Much less tendency for remission than in ulcerative colitis.
Effect of operation	Following colectomy, disease usually does not recur.	If terminal ileum is involved, fistulae and abscess occur following resection. Disease often recurs at or distal to anastomosis.
Toxic megacolon and perforation	Common	Rare
Cancer of colon	Twenty-five times as common as in same age group of general populations.	*Rare*, but the fact that these relatively young patients have resections earlier than those with ulcerative colitis may be a partial explanation.
Gross blood in stools	Common	Rare. If present, it almost always indicates disease in the *rectum* and *sigmoid*.
Arthritis, iritis, dermatitis	Common	Less common
Fistulae	Rare	Common

and pathological manifestations of both diseases. However, it is considered worthwhile to try to make the differential diagnosis, since about three-fourths of the cases will often have reasonably characteristic radiological features of one or the other disease. It must be emphasized that the correct diagnosis can be made in the vast majority of cases by properly correlating the clinical, radiological, and pathological changes (see summary of differential diagnostic features in Table 1).

In summary, although it may be impossible to differentiate some cases of ulcerative colitis and granulomatous colitis radiologically, clinically, and pathologically, the typical radiological appearances seen in this case are strongly in favor of ulcerative colitis. It is fortunate that with proper medical treatment many cases of acute ulcerative colitis are completely reversible, in contrast to the indolent progression of granulomatous colitis.

SUGGESTED READINGS

ULCERATIVE AND GRANULOMATOUS COLITIS

1. Kent TH, Ammon RK, DenBesten L: Differentiation of ulcerative colitis and regional enteritis of colon. Arch Pathol 89:20–29, 1970
2. Kirsner JB, Palmer WL, Klotz AP: Reversibility in ulcerative colitis. Radiology 57:1–14, 1951
3. Marshak RH, Lindner AE: Ulcerative and granulomatous colitis. In AR Margulis, HJ Burhenne: Alimentary Tract Roentgenology, Vol 2, pp 742–788. CV Mosby Co, St. Louis, 1967
4. Neschis M, Siegelman SS, Parker JG: Diagnosis and management of the megacolon of ulcerative colitis. Gastroenterology 55: 251–259, 1968
5. Reeves BF, Carlson HC, Dockerty MB: Segmental ulcerative colitis versus segmental Crohn's disease of the colon: a roentgenographic and pathologic study. Am J Roentgenol 99:24–34, 1967
6. Schachter H, Goldstein MJ, Rappaport H, Fennessy JJ, Kirsner JB: Ulcerative and "granulomatous" colitis: validity of differential diagnostic criteria. A study of 100 patients treated by total colectomy. Ann Intern Med 72:841–851, 1970
7. Stein GN, Roy RH, Finkelstein AK: Roentgen changes in ulcerative colitis. Semin in Roentgenol 3:3–26, 1968

ACUTE VASCULAR OCCLUSION

Schwartz S, Boley SJ, Robinson K, Krieger H, Schultz L, Allen AC: Roentgenologic features of vascular disorders of the intestines. Radiol Clin North Am 2: 71–87, 1964

AMEBIASIS

1. Reeder MM, Hamilton LC: Tropical diseases of the colon. Semin in Roentgenol *3:*62–80, 1968
2. Weinfeld A: The roentgen appearance of intestinal amebiasis. Am J Roentgenol *96:*311–322, 1966

CATHARTIC COLON

1. Dreyfus JR, Janower ML: The colon. In LL Robbins (ed): *Golden's Diagnostic Radiology, Section 5: Digestive Tract*, pp 921–922. Williams & Wilkins Co, Baltimore, 1969
2. Heilbrun N, Bernstein C: Roentgen abnormalities of the large and small intestine associated with prolonged cathartic ingestion. Radiology *65:*549–556, 1955

CORRECT ANSWERS

Question 1-(C)
Question 2-(B)
Question 3-(B)
Question 4-(C)
Question 5-(E)
Question 6-(E)

NOTES

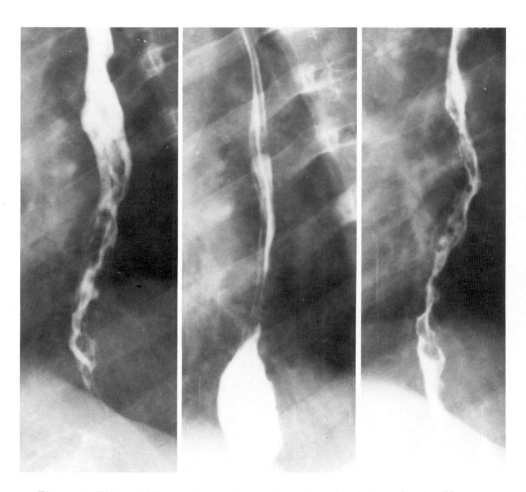

Figure 3. This middle-aged man has epigastric and substernal pain. You are shown three spot roentgenograms of the esophagus.

Questions 7 through 10

7. Which one of the following is the *MOST* likely diagnosis?

   (A) Monilial esophagitis
   (B) Esophageal varices
   (C) Carcinoma
   (D) Scleroderma
   (E) Reflux esophagitis

8. Which one of the following is *LEAST* characteristic of monilial esophagitis?

   (A) Pain
   (B) Associated debilitating systemic diseases
   (C) Oral involvement
   (D) Esophageal spasm
   (E) Hemorrhage

9. "Down-hill" varices occur in which one of the following conditions?

   (A) Obstruction of the superior vena cava
   (B) Obstruction of the portal vein
   (C) Obstruction of the inferior vena cava
   (D) Obstruction of the hepatic vein
   (E) None of the above

10. Which one of the following statements concerning esophageal carcinoma is *MOST* likely?

   (A) It most commonly occurs in the proximal one third
   (B) It is most often polypoid
   (C) Adenocarcinoma is the most common cell type
   (D) There is a higher incidence in achalasia
   (E) Lesions in the distal one third have the best prognosis

Discussion

The correct answer to question 7 is (B). The tortuous radiolucencies occupying the lumen of the distal few inches of the esophagus and the variability in their appearance on the three views are characteristic of varices. These views represent three successive "spot" roentgenograms made within a few moments of each other on one piece of 8- by 10-inch film. In the relaxed esophagus (Figure 3, *left view*) the varices are well shown, whereas the passage of a primary peristaltic wave caused them to disappear completely a few seconds later (Figure 3, *middle view*) by squeezing the blood from the varices through the veins in the wall of the esophagus into the periesophageal plexus. Conversely, when the esophagus again relaxes (Figure 3, *right view*) there is, again, enough space in the lumen to allow refilling of the varices. The technique for demonstrating varices will be discussed later.

Monilial esophagitis shows a ragged unchanging contour of the esophageal mucosa with multiple tiny indentations and protrusions, most of which are probably tiny undermined ulcers. As a result of this appearance this disease has sometimes been termed "intramural diverticulosis of the esophagus". In some cases of moniliasis the esophagus is covered with a thick pseudomembrane, whereas in others the granular friable edematous mucosa contains many tiny ulcers which cause the characteristic "fuzzy" or ragged appearance. The shape, caliber, and ragged mucosal surface do not change appreciably during the examination in moniliasis, thus differing from the rapidly changing roentgen appearance of esophageal varices as shown here. It is also characteristic for varices to be invisible if there is too much barium in the lumen (Figure 3A) or after the esophagus contracts and squeezes the blood out of the varices (Figure 3, *middle view*). Conversely, in moniliasis the peristalsis is very sluggish or absent in the involved areas of the esophagus and the esophageal lumen is frequently narrowed due to the associated spasm, pseudomembrane, and marked inflammatory edema of the wall of the esophagus.

Although most esophageal carcinomas are of the relatively short annular type, there is the rare so-called "varicoid carcinoma" which will occasionally involve a longer segment. In such an unusual carcinoma the multiple polypoid intrusions into the lumen might, at first glance, simulate large esophageal varices. However, the virtually *constant* configuration of such a carcinoma on multiple views and the relatively abrupt transition between the

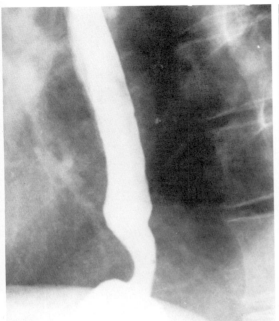
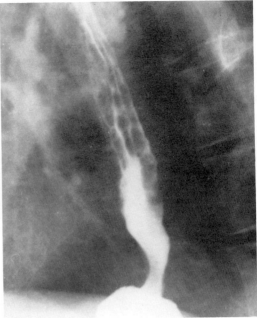

Figure 3A   Figure 3B

normal portions of the esophagus and the lesion itself should alert the radiologist to the correct diagnosis of a rigid nodular lesion; i.e., a carcinoma.

Scleroderma is characterized primarily by diminished or absent primary peristaltic waves in an esophagus with a lumen of normal or greater-than-normal caliber. Furthermore, there are no intraluminal mucosal lesions such as are present with varices or carcinoma and none of the intramural ulcers, rigidity, or spasm as seen in moniliasis.

Reflux esophagitis is usually, but not always, associated with a sliding type of gastric hiatal hernia which is not present in this case. This type of esophagitis may occur in association with destruction of the squamous epithelium lining the lower esophagus and often causes a fuzzy serrated appearance of the mucosa above the hernia. The destruction of the squamous epithelium lining the lower esophagus is often followed by an upward overgrowth of the columnar epithelium from the gastric cardia ("Barrett's esophagus"). If the denuded, chronically inflamed surface is not covered by the columnar epithelium, strictures may develop. These are usually 4 or 5 cm. above the cardioesophageal junction.

QUESTION 8

Dysphagia and episodes of substernal pain are caused by the segmental spasm which frequently occurs in moniliasis. Hemorrhage has *not* been re-

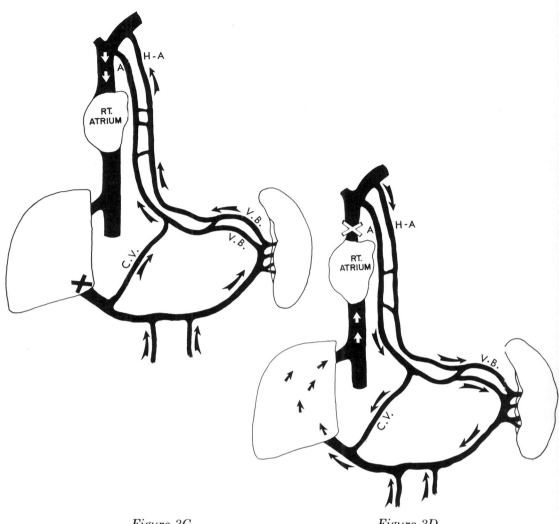

Figure 3C   Figure 3D

ported in this disease. Therefore, **the correct answer to question 8 is (E)**. Moniliasis may be associated with oral involvement ("thrush"), although the latter may not always be present. Although moniliasis may rarely occur in a relatively healthy patient, it is almost always seen in patients with debilitating systemic diseases such as leukemia, or in patients under treatment with immunosuppressive drugs, antibiotics, or steroids.

QUESTION 9

Most cases of varices are of the "uphill" type (Figure 3C, *black arrows*) seen in hepatic cirrhosis in which disease there is intrahepatic obstruction ("X" in Figure 3C) to the flow of blood from the portal venous system. Since much of the portal blood cannot get through the liver and thence into the inferior vena cava and back to the heart, it must go *via* another route which nature has provided in the form of the coronary vein ("*C.V.*" in Figure 3C) and vasa brevia ("*V.B.*" in Figure 3C). The portal blood flows from these veins through the esophagogastric hiatus into the periesophageal plexus which, in turn, communicates *via* veins in the wall of the esophagus with the venous plexus in the submucosa of the esophagus and gastric cardia. Blood from the periesophageal plexus flows into the azygos ("*A*" in Figure 3C) and hemiazygos ("*H-A*" in Figure 3C) system and enters the superior vena cava through which it flows (Figure 3C, *white arrows*) into the right atrium. Thus, by this circuitous collateral route the portal blood reaches the heart. Conversely, when venous blood from the head and upper extremities cannot reach the heart owing to an obstruction ("*X*" in Figure 3D) of the superior vena cava, it, too, must find an alternative route to the heart (Figure 3D). In the event that the superior vena cava is occluded at the level of the azygos entrance to the vena cava, the highest intercostal veins provide a communication between the branches of the brachiocephalic venous trunks and the azygos-hemiazygos and internal mammary systems of veins. The large amount of venous blood from the head and upper extremities then must flow downward through the azygos ("*A*" in Figure 3D) and hemiazygos ("*H-A*" in Figure 3D) system since it cannot reach the heart owing to the occlusion of the superior vena cava. It thus flows "downhill" (Figure 3D) through the azygos-hemiazygos system, the periesophageal plexus, the coronary veins, and eventually enters the portal vein. It then passes from the intrahepatic portal venous system and the hepatic vein to reach the inferior vena cava through which it flows (*white arrows*, Figure 3D) to reach the right atrium.

It is understandable that the large volume of blood which flows through the esophageal plexus under these circumstances would result in the formation of esophageal varices. By now you have correctly concluded that such varices are called "downhill" varices (Figure 3D) because the direction of blood flow through them is *downward* toward the liver, in contrast to the reversed direction of the flow of blood in "uphill" varices. Therefore, **the correct answer to question 9 is (A).**

Extrahepatic obstruction of the portal vein, the hepatic vein (Budd-Chiari syndrome) or the inferior vena cava above the entrance of the hepatic vein would result in the development of the much more common "uphill" varices, the most frequent cause of which is the type of intrahepatic obstruction associated with cirrhosis of the liver. Obstruction of the inferior vena cava below the level of the hepatic vein would not result in esophageal varices, although such an obstruction could result in the development of ureteral vein varices if the obstruction is located above the renal veins.

QUESTION 10

The correct answer to question 10 is (E); i.e., carcinomas which involve the distal one third of the esophagus have the best prognosis, whereas those more proximally located often involve vital mediastinal structures such as aorta, vena cava, and left main stem bronchus, which may preclude complete resection. All other possible answers listed are incorrect; i.e., carcinomas are more common in the distal one third of the esophagus than in the more proximal portions, and they are usually annular in type, rather than polypoid. The most common cell type is squamous carcinoma. There is no convincing evidence that there is a higher incidence of carcinoma in patients with achalasia.

DISCUSSION

Once esophageal varices have been demonstrated on roentgenograms or cine studies, they are readily recognized. However, their demonstration is not always easy and is dependent upon several important factors. The two most important technical requirements are (1) a *small amount* of barium in the lumen (Figure 3, *right and left views*, and Figure 3B) and (2) a *relaxed* esophagus (Figure 3, *right and left views*, and Figure 3B). Normally, if a patient swallows only *once* the esophagus will remain contracted for 10 to 30 seconds following the passage of the primary peristaltic wave initiated by that single swallow. The appearance of the contracted esophagus after the passage of the primary wave is well seen (Figure 3, *middle view*). When the esophagus is contracted there is no space in the lumen for the varices and they cannot fill with blood. The blood in the submucosal varices in the relaxed esophagus (Figure 3, *left view*) will be squeezed out (Figure 3, *middle view*) through the intramural veins which communicate with the periesophageal plexus, and the varices will not be apparent. Conversely, when the esophagus relaxes, the blood can again flow into the submucosal varices which now have space to fill and will thus project into the lumen where a *small amount* of barium will show them (Figure 3, *right view*). Varices will often be completely *obscured* if there is too much barium in the lumen (Figure 3A), whereas a few seconds later with smaller amounts of barium in a relaxed esophagus, the varices are easily shown (Figure 3B).

In order to achieve relaxation of the esophagus following the passage of a primary wave, it is important that the patient *refrain from swallowing* after one bolus of barium is swallowed, because each succeeding swallow initiates another primary peristaltic wave which will progress through the already contracted esophagus, thus resulting in another continued contraction. However, if the patient is able to refrain from swallowing (not always an easy thing for patients), no further primary peristaltic wave will be initiated and the contracted esophagus will eventually relax. If thick barium has been administered and some has adhered to the mucosa after the passage of the primary wave (Figure 3, *middle view*), the varices will usually show when the esophagus relaxes (Figure 3, *right view*). For those patients who have difficulty in refraining from swallowing, the sustained performance of the Valsalva maneuver will *preclude* further swallowing, thus *preventing* the initiation of further primary peristaltic waves while the radiologist waits for the esophagus to relax. Probably the most important reason for performing the Valsalva maneuver is to bring about relaxation of the esophagus.

During the Valsalva maneuver it may also be possible to cause *reflux* of small amounts of barium from the phrenic ampulla (Figure 3, *middle view*) into the esophagus as it relaxes (Figure 3, *right view*). Thus, the sustained performance of the Valsalva maneuver immediately after a swallow of barium is a good way to cause a *small* amount of barium to flow retrograde from the phrenic ampulla into the esophageal lumen. This is a valuable maneuver to try in those patients in whom the first primary wave has a tendency to "strip" the mucosa clean of the barium.

In summary, it is, admittedly, not always easy to cause the esophagus to *relax* and it is not always easy to get a small amount of barium to remain in the relaxed lumen. However, the examiner will do well to remember that he is trying to achieve a condition in which a *relaxed* esophagus contains a *small amount of barium*. If he knows how to direct his energies and skills toward achieving this situation he will have the best chance of showing varices.

SUGGESTED READINGS

ESOPHAGEAL VARICES

1. Brombart M: Roentgenology of the esophagus. In AR Margulis, HJ Burhenne: *Alimentary Tract Roentgenology*, Vol 1, pp 301–305. CV Mosby Co, St Louis, 1967.
2. Nelson SW: The roentgenologic diagnosis of esophageal varices. Am J Roentgenol *77:*599–611, 1957
3. Felson B, Lessure AP: "Downhill" varices of esophagus. Dis Chest *46:*740–746, 1964
4. Mikkelsen WJ: Varices of the upper esophagus in superior vena caval obstruction. Radiology *81:*945–948, 1963

MONILIAL ESOPHAGITIS

1. Andren L, Theander G: Roentgenographic appearances of esophageal moniliasis. Acta Radiol *46:*571–574, 1956
2. Sanders E, Levinthal C, Donner MW: Monilia esophagitis in a patient with

hemoglobin SC disease: demonstration of esophageal motor abnormality by cine-radiofluorography. Ann Intern Med *57:*650–654, 1962

3. Troupin RH: Intramural esophageal diverticulosis and moniliasis: a possible association. Am J Roentgenol *104:*613–616, 1968

4. Hodes PJ, Atkins JP, Hodes BL: Esophageal intramural diverticulosis. Am J Roentgenol *96:*411–413, 1966

REFLUX ESOPHAGITIS

Sandry RJ: The pathology of chronic oesophagitis. Gut *3:* 189–200, 1962

CORRECT ANSWERS

Question 7-(B)
Question 8-(E)
Question 9-(A)
Question 10-(E)

NOTES

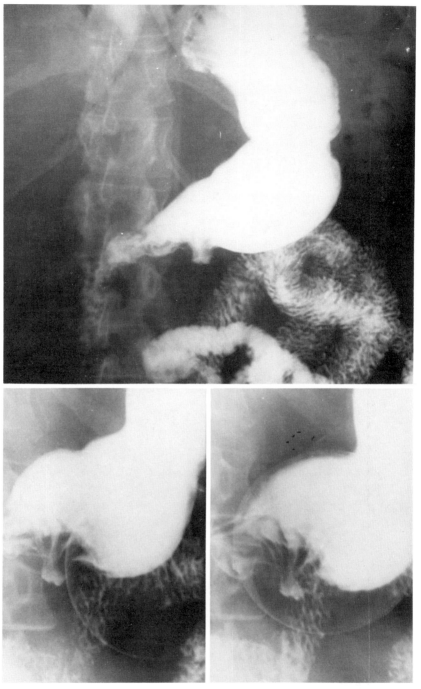

Figures 4 (top), 5 (lower left), and 6 (lower right). This 48-year-old woman has weight loss, vomiting, and epigastric pain. Figure 4 is a posteroanterior roentgenogram of the stomach, and Figures 5 and 6 are spot roentgenograms of the stomach.

Questions 11 through 14

11. Which one of the following is the *MOST* likely diagnosis?
    (A) Benign gastric ulcer
    (B) Ulcerated carcinoma
    (C) Ulcerated leiomyoma
    (D) Diverticulum
    (E) Ulcerated lymphoma

12. Which one of the following roentgenographic signs is *MOST* suggestive of a benign ulcer?
    (A) Penetration beyond the gastric wall
    (B) Crater less than 3 cm. in diameter
    (C) Meniscus sign
    (D) Lesser curvature location
    (E) Abrupt transition between normal gastric mucosa and mound of tissue which surrounds the crater

13. Which one of the following roentgenographic signs is *MOST* suggestive of a malignant ulcer?
    (A) Greater curvature location
    (B) Antral location
    (C) Carman's sign
    (D) Hampton's line
    (E) Smooth mound of tissue around the ulcer

14. Which one of the following statements concerning gastric diverticula is *INCORRECT*?
    (A) Congenital (true) gastric diverticula are considered to be incomplete duplications
    (B) Most gastric diverticula are located on the posterior wall of the cardia near the lesser curvature
    (C) The most common complication is hemorrhage
    (D) Acquired (false) diverticula are usually located near the pylorus
    (E) Gastric diverticula have a tendency to empty rapidly

Discussion

QUESTION 11

The most likely diagnosis here is benign gastric ulcer, and **the correct answer to question 11 is (A).** Illustrations of the compression spot films (Figures 6B and C) show the gastric mucosal folds radiating to the very *edge* of the crater. Note also that this crater projects beyond the *expected margin of the lumen* (Figures 6A, B, and C, *broken lines*).* The radiation of folds into the crater and the penetration beyond the lumen are probably the two signs which are most suggestive of benignancy. By careful scrutiny one will also see a tiny "polypoid" defect in the base of the crater (*arrows in Figures 6B and C*). This is a blood clot which now occludes the small artery which had bled prior to the examination. There is also a mound of smoothly defined tissue (Figure 6A, *arrows*) around the crater, this being the so-called "ulcer mound" (see also Figures 6L, M, and N, *arrows*). The smooth surface of the mound and its imperceptible transition with the normal gastric wall both proximally and distally strongly suggest a zone of edema around a benign ulcer.

It may be difficult or impossible to differentiate ulcerated carcinomas from benign gastric ulcers on the basis of roentgenographic findings. However, in contrast to the smooth mound of edematous tissue around a benign ulcer, the mound of neoplastic tissue surrounding a malignant ulcer is usually nodular (Figure 6R, *black arrows*), and the transition between this neoplastic tissue and the normal gastric wall is usually rather *abrupt* (Figure 6E, *arrows on the left side,* and Figure 6R, *white arrow*). Furthermore, ulcerated carcinomas do not penetrate beyond the normal gastric lumen, but are usually located within it (Figure 6R), since the ulcer is merely a necrotic area in the relatively *flat* thin intraluminal mass (*arrows* in Figure 6E).

Although most leiomyomas are easily recognized intraluminal *polypoid* masses, occasionally such tumors may be almost entirely extramural. Should an ulcer be present in the small, poorly defined, intramural portion of such a lesion, it might, at first glance, resemble the benign crater shown here, particularly if the crater were well circumscribed ("punched out") However, the large extramural mass of such a leiomyoma can usually be recognized, because it produces an indentation of the gastric wall from which it arises. The crater in such a lesion is located in the center of the indented area. There is no evidence of such an extramural mass in the case shown here.

* The broken lines in the subsequent illustrations in this case indicate the expected margin of the lumen.

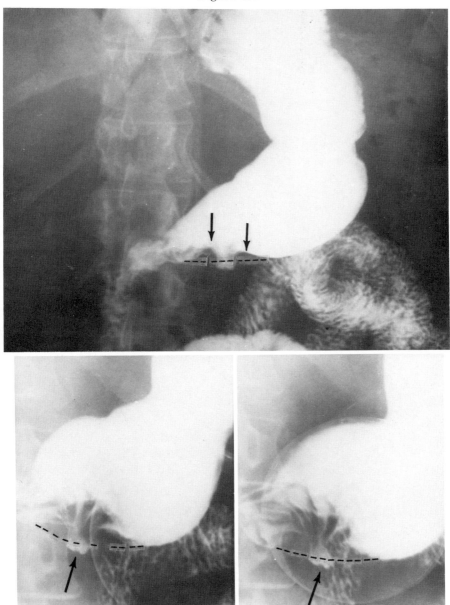

Figure 6B   *Figure 6C*

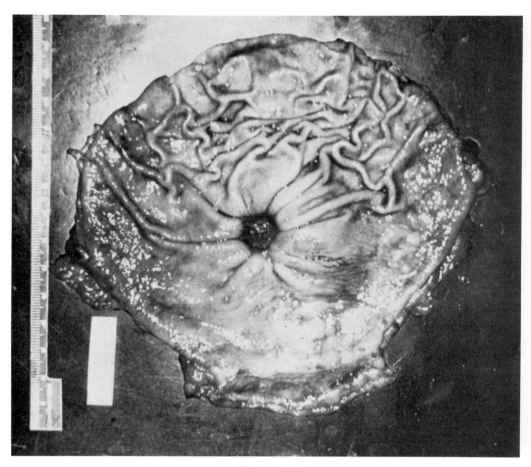

Figure 6D

True congenital gastric diverticula occur on the posterior wall of the cardia close to the esophagocardiac junction, but do not occur in the antrum. They do not have the rather square configuration of the typical benign ulcer shown here, but instead have the narrow neck leading into the sac-like diverticulum. Other gastric diverticula are *acquired* as the result of postoperative scarring or inflammatory disease, and are usually located in the region of the pylorus where they are termed "pseudodiverticula". The history of pyloroplasty and the inflammatory type of deformity of the gastric antrum, pylorus, and duodenal bulb should provide the clue to the correct diagnosis of such "pseudodiverticula".

In an ulcerated lymphoma, as in an ulcerated carcinoma, there is often a nodular irregular surface of the tissue surrounding the crater, in contrast to the smooth mound of edematous tissue shown here. Furthermore, as is true in ulcerated carcinomas, there is often an abrupt transition between the

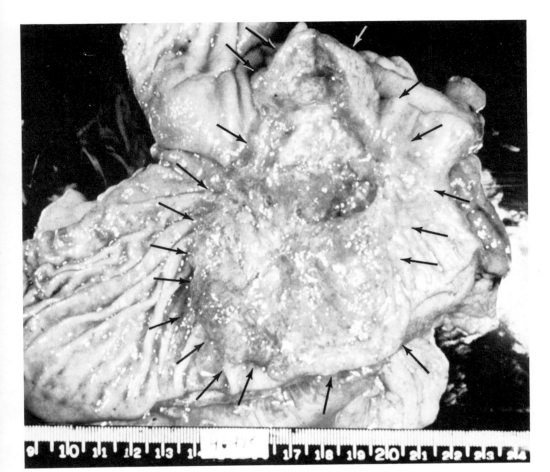

Figure 6E

lymphomatous tissue and the adjacent normal gastric tissue. Since none of these signs of malignancy is present in the illustrations shown here, lymphoma would not be likely.

QUESTION 12

Of all the roentgenographic signs mentioned in question 12 **the one which is most suggestive of a benign ulcer is (A),** i.e., *penetration* beyond the gastric wall (Figures 6F, G, I, and J). The size and location of a crater are of very little differential diagnostic value. The meniscus sign of Carman (Figures 6O, P, and Q) is not suggestive of benignancy, but is diagnostic of a specific type of ulcerated carcinoma which will be discussed later. As stated previously, *nodularity* of the tissue surrounding the crater and an *abrupt transition* between the normal gastric mucosa and this irreg-

Figure 6F

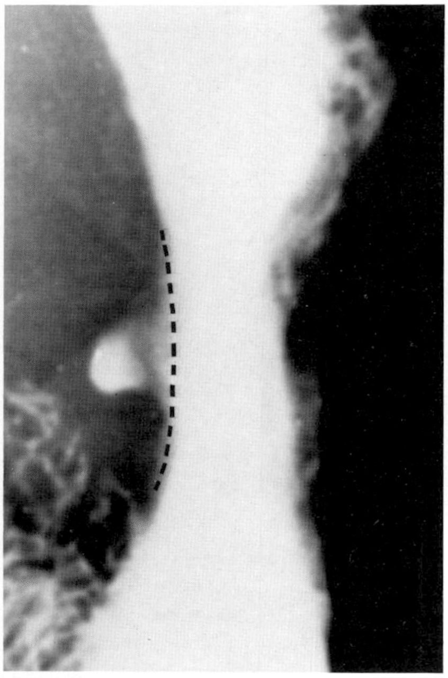

Figure 6G

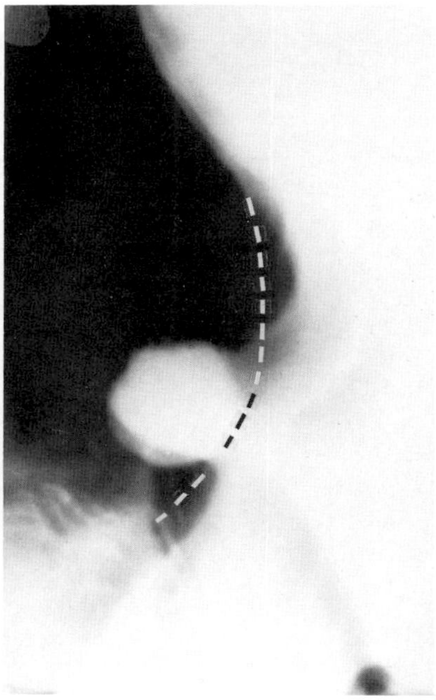

Figure 6H

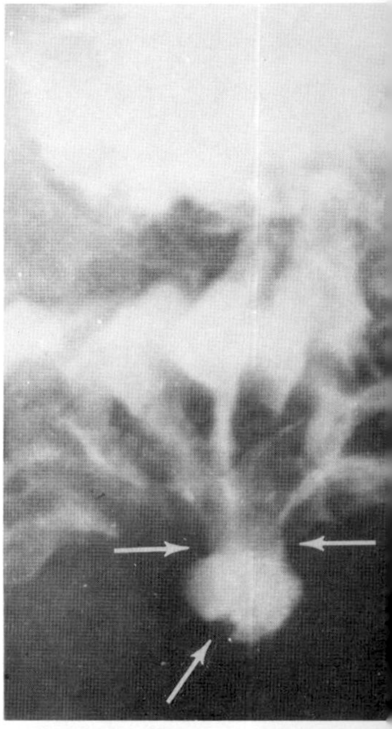

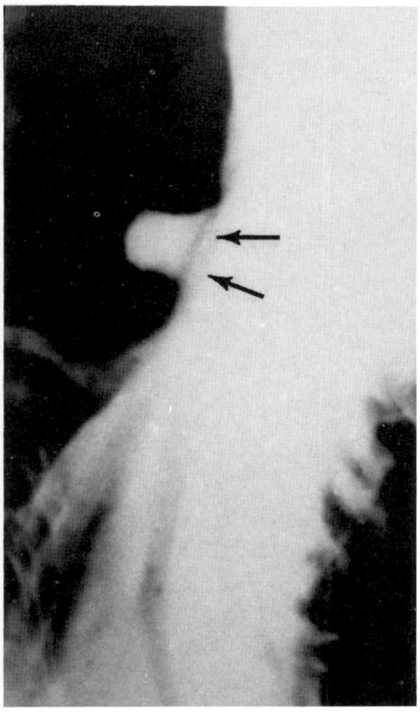

Figure 6I

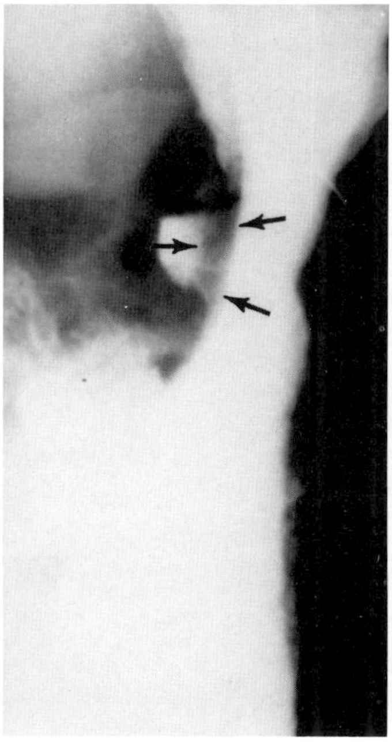

Figure 6J

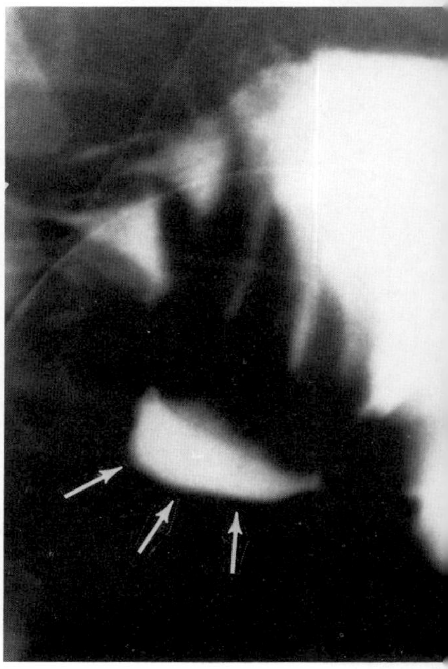

Figure 6K

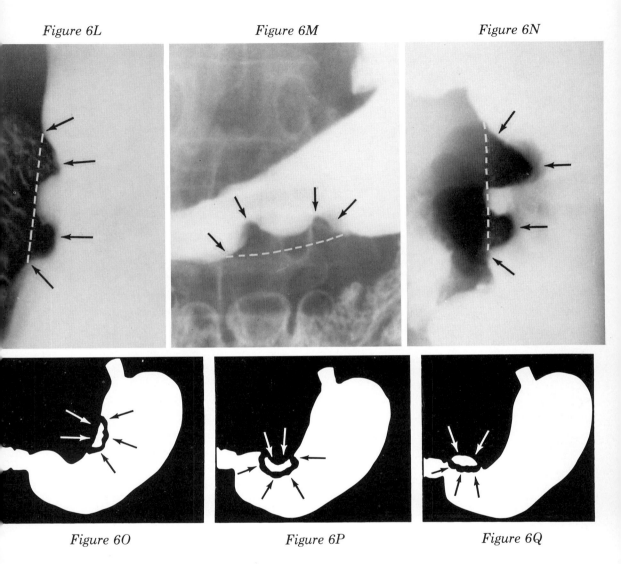

Figure 6L

Figure 6M

Figure 6N

Figure 6O

Figure 6P

Figure 6Q

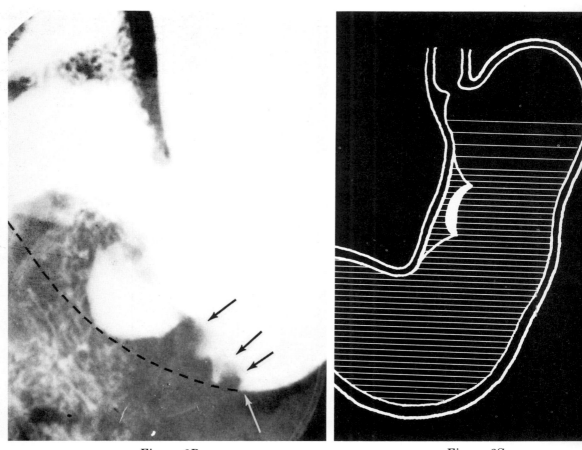

| Figure 6R | Figure 6S |

ular mound of tissue are the roentgen findings which would favor the diagnosis of an ulcerated neoplasm, as opposed to the characteristic roentgen signs of benign ulcer which are demonstrated in this case.

QUESTION 13

The correct answer to question 13 is (C). Of the findings listed in this question, the one which is most suggestive of a malignant ulcer is Carman's meniscus sign (see Figures 47 and 48, p. 224). This is a reliable sign, and although there are various interpretations of Carman's description and diagram (Figure 6S), the sign is virtually diagnostic of the *specific* type of malignant neoplasm with which it is associated. The sign actually refers to the *profiled* configuration (Figures 6O, P, and Q) of the barium trapped by the compression and resulting folding together of the opposite edges of the elevated rim of the neoplastic tissue which forms the margin of this unusual and *specific* type of neoplasm. The *base* (outer margin) of the barium collection trapped in such a lesion is almost always located where the *expected* normal gastric wall would be (*white arrows* in Figures 6O, P, and Q), since there is relatively little intraluminal mass associated with this specific type of neoplasm, except for the elevated rim of tissue at the periphery of the lesion. It is worth remembering that the *inner* margin of the trapped barium collection is *always convex toward the lumen* (Figures 6O, P, and Q). The gastric wall forming the base of the Carman type of lesion is minimally thickened and fibrotic, in contrast to the elevated intraluminal rim at the periphery of the lesion where there is more rapid growth of the carcinoma because of its proximity to a more normal blood supply in the adjacent normal gastric wall. When the somewhat circular rim of a Carman type of carcinoma is folded by compression, the displacement of the barium by the apposed halves of the rim produces a somewhat *semicircular* intraluminal curvilinear radiolucency (*black arrows* in Figures 6O, P, and Q) paralleling the inner (luminal) margin of the aforementioned trapped barium collection. Note that all of these trapped barium collections are in the shape of a lens ("meniscus"), one being plano-convex (Figure 6O), one concavoconvex (Figure 6P), and one biconvex (Figure 6Q). The inner aspect is always convex toward the lumen (see Figures 47 and 48, p. 224).

The location of a crater on the greater curvature is *not* indicative of an ulcerated neoplasm since the majority of these craters are benign (Figure 6H). Neither is the location in the antrum helpful in arriving at a diagnosis of malignant ulcer. Hampton's line is never seen in an ulcerated neoplasm, but is virtually diagnostic of a *benign* ulcer, since it indicates peptic digestion of the submucosa beneath an overhanging edge of relatively nonedematous mucosa, which, when seen in profile, appears as a fine radiolucent line (Figure 6I) at the base of the crater due to the displacement of the barium by this thin rim, or "washer", of tissue which overhangs the mouth of the crater. As stated previously, the smooth surface of the mound of tissue around the ulcer shown here is suggestive of a benign lesion rather than a malignant one.

QUESTION 14

Since gastric diverticula empty slowly, **the correct answer to question 14 is (E).** Most gastric diverticula occur high on the posterior wall of the stomach in the region of the cardia close to the esophagogastric junction, and since they usually have a narrow neck leading into the redundant sac-like diverticulum, they have a tendency to retain barium for several hours whether the patient is erect or recumbent. All of the other statements about gastric diverticula are *true* and, therefore, should not be considered, since you were looking for the *incorrect* statement.

By comparing the gross specimen of the benign ulcer illustrated here (Figure 6D) with that of a similar case of an ulcerated neoplasm (Figure 6E) one can immediately see the differences in the appearance of the benign ulcer mound and the mound of neoplastic tissue. The benign ulcer mound is smooth, and its transition with normal mucosa is so gradual as to be imperceptible (Figures 6D and A), whereas the surface of the neoplastic tissue is nodular (Figure 6E, and Figure 6R, *black arrows*) and irregular without evidence of mucosal folds. There is also a point of *abrupt* transition between normal and neoplastic tissue (Figure 6E, *arrows on the left*, and Figure 6R, *white arrow*). These findings clearly help to explain the radiographic appearance of such a lesion.

Other signs of benignancy are those related to the *undermining* of the mucosa owing to the fact that it is more resistant to peptic digestion than is the submucosa which is destroyed at a more rapid rate. Thus, the more resistant, *less* rapidly destroyed mucosa overhangs the *more* rapidly destroyed submucosa. If the overhanging mucosa is *minimally* edematous, a thin black line (Hampton's line) is seen at the base of the perfectly profiled crater (*arrows* in Figure 6I) corresponding to the displacement of the barium by the tangentially oriented thin "washer" of overhanging mucosa. If the undermined mucosa is *more edematous*, a wider radiolucent line termed the "ulcer collar" (Figure 6J, *between arrows*) is seen when the crater is viewed in profile, because the thicker "washer" of edematous overhanging mucosal tissue displaces more barium. Undermining of the mucosa also helps to explain one of the clichés so frequently quoted about benign ulcers i.e., they are often "collar-button" shaped (Figure 6H). The overhanging mucosa may be enormously edematous and can almost occlude the orifice of certain benign craters, causing interesting crescent-shaped barium collections (Figure 6K) to be trapped in their bases. This configuration of the trapped barium is probably a fairly diagnostic sign of a benign crater. Interestingly enough, this sign is often first noted when oral cholecystographic contrast material is trapped in the depths of the greatly undermined crater the entrance to which is partly obstructed by the markedly edematous overhanging mucosa. Thus, the sign may be first noted during attempts to study the gallbladder *prior* to the upper gastrointestinal examination. It is also of interest that this so-called "crescent sign", which indicates a benign type of lesion, is similar in appearance to Carman's mysterious "Figure 4" (Figure 6S) because the *inner* margin of the crescent-shaped barium collection diagrammed in Carman's figure is also *concave toward* the lumen, whereas the outer margin is *convex away* from the lumen. However, by careful analysis of Carman's article one can reason that the roentgenologic sign of the specific type of carcinoma which he so clearly described can only be manifested by a barium collection, which, when profiled, has its *convexity* directed *toward the lumen*, its outer margin corresponding to the expected margin of the gastric wall (Figures 6-O, P, and Q, and Figures 47 and 48, p. 224). Furthermore, the barium trapped in the Carman type of carcinoma is always *intraluminal*, in contrast to the frequent *extraluminal* location of the "crescent sign" of benign gastric ulcer.

The vast majority of gastric ulcers are benign (more than 95 per cent in most series) and most will heal completely during medical therapy. The typical benign ulcer will ordinarily diminish to one half or less of its original size in 2 or 3 weeks and some will show complete healing in this period of time. If an ulcer does not completely heal in 6 weeks, it is *doubtful* that it will heal with a longer period of medical management. This is probably due to the fact that the poorly vascularized fibrous tissue in the base does not favor complete healing. Even though such lesions are clearly benign from the roentgen standpoint, they represent a threat to the patient's life owing to the danger of hemorrhage or perforation during subsequent enlargement. Thus, if it is not possible to follow a patient with serial roentgen studies to confirm healing, some surgeons believe it is advisable to consider resection at the outset.

About 50 to 60 per cent of gastric ulcers can be accurately diagnosed on the basis of reliable roentgenographic signs of benignancy or malignancy. Those in which such roentgenographic signs cannot be demonstrated should be termed "indeterminate". Although the vast majority of such indeterminate lesions are benign, they are best studied by careful follow-up to confirm prompt healing, as mentioned previously. Since the radiographic criteria for benignancy of gastric ulcers are quite reliable, and since the incidence of malignancy will usually not exceed 3 to 5 per cent of all gastric ulcers, it seems reasonable to disagree with those who advocate surgical treatment of *all* gastric ulcers. Furthermore, the mortality rate from gastric resection may approach that which is ascribed to errors in the early roentgenologic diagnosis of malignancy.

SUGGESTED READINGS

GASTRIC ULCER

1. Nelson SW: The discovery of gastric ulcers and the differential diagnosis between benignancy and malignancy. Radiol Clin North Am 7:5–25, 1969
2. Nelson SW: A crescent-shaped collection of residual cholecystographic contrast material: a new sign of benign gastric ulcer? Am J Roentgenol *116:* 293–303, 1972

3. Wolf BS: Observation on roentgen features of benign and malignant gastric ulcers. Semin in Roentgenol 6:140–150, 1971
4. Wolf BS, Marshak RH: Profile features of benign gastric niches on roentgen examination. J Mount Sinai Hosp New York 24:604–626, 1957
5. Wolf BS, Sherkow CJ: Carman sign of ulcerating gastric carcinoma. Am J Digest Dis 2:467–477, 1957
6. Zboralske FF: Gastric ulcer. In AR Margulis, HJ Burhenne: *Alimentary Tract Roentgenology, Vol 1*, pp 475–487. CV Mosby Co, St Louis, 1967

CORRECT ANSWERS

Question 11-(A)
Question 12-(A)
Question 13-(C)
Question 14-(E)

NOTES

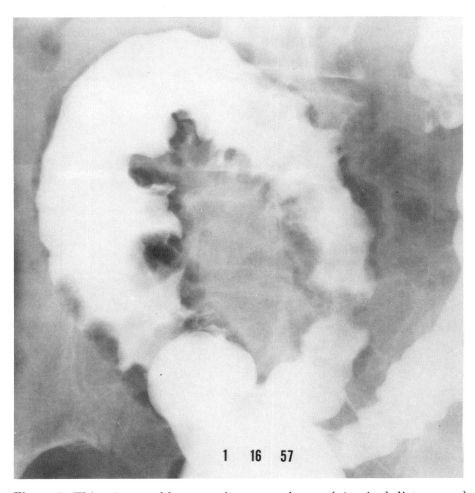

1 16 57

Figure 7. This 48-year-old woman has vague lower abdominal distress and constipation. You are shown a view of the barium-filled sigmoid.

Questions 15 through 19

15. Which one of the following is the *MOST* likely diagnosis?

    (A) Multiple adenomatous polyps
    (B) Colitis cystica profunda
    (C) Pseudopolyps of granulomatous colitis
    (D) Pneumatosis cystoides intestinalis
    (E) Acute vascular occlusion

16. Which one of the following statements concerning adenomatous polyps of the colon is *MOST* likely?

    (A) They are usually benign if pedunculated
    (B) They are more common in the proximal than in the distal colon
    (C) Pedunculated and sessile polyps have the same incidence of malignancy
    (D) An increase in size indicates malignancy
    (E) Lesions 2 cm. or larger are usually malignant

17. Which one of the following statements is *LEAST* characteristic of colitis cystica profunda?

    (A) It occurs primarily in the lower part of the colon
    (B) The cysts commonly contain mucus
    (C) The cysts are numerous
    (D) It is primarily a disease of adults
    (E) It is a precancerous condition

18. Which one of the following disorders is *MOST* commonly associated with pneumatosis cystoides intestinalis?

    (A) Constipation
    (B) Infection of the wall of the colon
    (C) Obstructive bronchopulmonary disease
    (D) Vascular insufficiency
    (E) Volvulus

19. Which one of the following statements concerning acute vascular occlusion of the colon is *LEAST* likely?

   (A) The sigmoid colon is the most common site
   (B) It may be reversible with complete return to normal
   (C) It may result in mucosal ulceration with subsequent stricture formation
   (D) It may result in necrosis and perforation
   (E) An arteriogram is helpful in confirming the diagnosis

Discussion

QUESTION 15

The correct answer to question 15 is (D). This case of pneumatosis cystoides intestinalis (pneumatosis coli) is shown to emphasize the importance of careful observation as well as differential diagnostic acumen. If you have not seen such a case before, it is understandable how you may have missed the diagnosis. After having seen this example you will be aware of the condition and remember the importance of carefully looking for the intramural "gas cysts" when you see multiple "polypoid" lesions in the sigmoid colon. Note that the "polypoid" lesions which indent the barium column in the sigmoid (Figure 7) have an appearance which, at first glance, might raise several diagnostic possibilities including multiple adenomatous polyps, the pseudopolyps associated with ulcerative and granulomatous types of colitis, and the "thumbprinting" seen in acute vascular occlusion of the sigmoid colon. However, in the case shown here the radiolucencies which indent the barium have *gas* density as proven by the fact that their *outer* margins (*arrows* in Figure 7A) are clearly demarcated from the adjacent water-density tissues. Such an appearance is diagnostic of the interesting condition termed pneumatosis coli or "pneumatosis cystoides intestinalis" of the colon. In this disease there are multiple gas-containing cysts of various sizes located most commonly in the subserosa, but sometimes in the submucosa. The overlying mucosa is entirely normal, as is the muscularis. Water-density lesions such as polyps, intramural hemorrhage ("thumbprinting"), and "pseudopolyps" can all be excluded once the gaseous density of the "polyps" has been noted. However, if you did *not* notice that these polypoid indentations of the intraluminal barium were due to gas cysts, it might be well to briefly consider the other roentgenological and clinical features which might help to exclude most of the other water-density lesions which were included as possible answers in question 15. First of all, it would be unlikely that multiple adenomatous polyps of the colon would be so numerous, so sessile, and so localized to the sigmoid. Colitis cystica profunda might be a possibility, but it is an unusual condition which is much less common than pneumatosis cystoides intestinalis. Furthermore, the patient whose roentgenogram is illustrated here was virtually asymptomatic, whereas colitis cystica is an inflammatory condition which usually produces rectal symptoms.

Chronic granulomatous colitis with "pseudopolyps" might be considered, but pseudopolyps as large as those shown here would be unlikely and the lumen of the rectum and sigmoid would probably be constricted by the time granulomatous colitis had progressed to the stage of so-called "cobblestoning" (see "cobblestoning" between the transverse ulcer indicated by the *small arrows* in Figure 36B). Furthermore, there are none of the transverse or longitudinal fissures or ulcers which are so characteristic of granulomatous colitis (see Figure 36B, *black arrows*).

Acute vascular occlusion with so-called "thumbprinting" due to intramural hemorrhage would, at first glance, seem like a reasonably good possibility, because the indentations of the barium column seen here do appear like "thumbprinting" (see medial aspect of cecum and ascending colon in Figure 27). However, an acute vascular occlusion severe enough to produce the extensive changes seen here would be associated with a more acute clinical picture than that manifested by the patient whose roentgenogram is illustrated here.

QUESTION 16

The correct answer to question 16 is (A); i.e., virtually all pedunculated polyps of the colon are benign. Probably two thirds (or more) of the colon polyps occur in the sigmoid and rectum. Sessile polyps have a much higher incidence of malignancy than do the pedunculated variety. However, although a recognizable increase in size is worrisome, it does not necessarily indicate a malignant lesion. Furthermore, although lesions more than 2 cm. in diameter have a higher incidence of malignancy, a sizeable number prove to be benign, particularly if they are pedunculated. Conversely, sessile lesions greater than 2 cm. in diameter have a higher incidence of malignancy than do those which have pedicles.

QUESTION 17

The correct answer to question 17 is (E), because colitis cystica profunda is *not* a precancerous condition. All the other statements listed as possible answers in this question are true and characteristic of this disease.

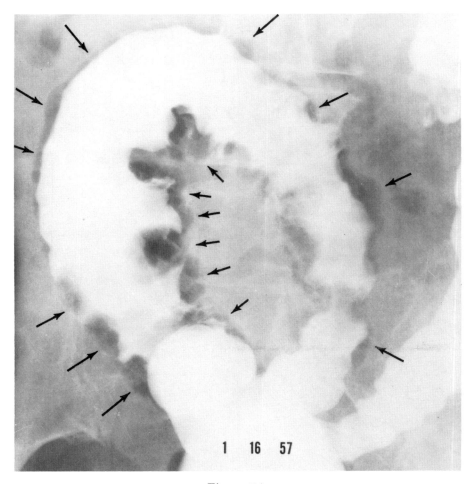

Figure 7A

QUESTION 18

The correct answer to question 18 is (C). Pneumatosis cystoides intestinalis of the colon in adults, as shown here, is frequently associated with obstructive bronchopulmonary disease. Infection of the wall of the colon, vascular insufficiency, and volvulus may also be associated with gas in the wall of the colon, but in these conditions the patient's clinical condition is much more serious than that of the patient whose roentgenograms are illustrated here. Furthermore, in sigmoid volvulus the sigmoid would probably not fill and the barium column would probably terminate in a "bird beak" deformity characteristic of volvulus. There would probably also be a greater degree of distention of the sigmoid. When intramural gas collections are associated with infection, occlusive vascular disease, or volvulus, the gas

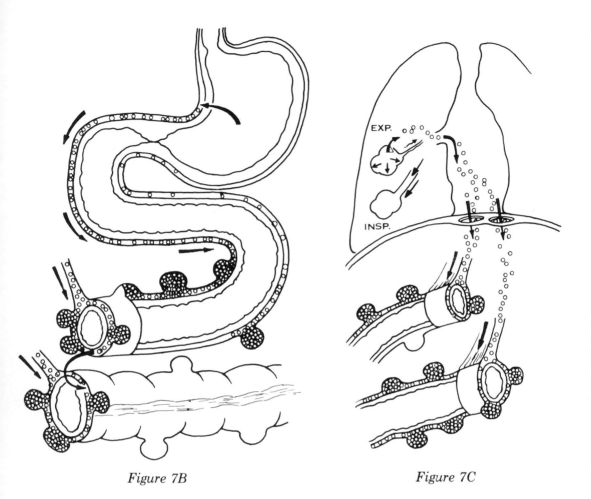

Figure 7B   Figure 7C

collections are almost always linear rather than cystic as we have illustrated here. Constipation is a nondiagnostic, nonspecific symptom which
has no proven relationship to pneumatosis coli.

QUESTION 19

The correct answer to question 19 is (A) because the roentgen
changes of acute vascular occlusion are *less* commonly seen in the sigmoid
colon and rectum than in the descending colon and the right side of the colon. This is probably related to the rich collateral blood supply from the inferior and middle hemorrhoidal arteries which anastomose with the superior
hemorrhoidal system of the inferior mesenteric artery.

Since all other possible answers listed in question 19 are *true*, they are all
incorrect answers. Acute vascular occlusion involving any part of the colon

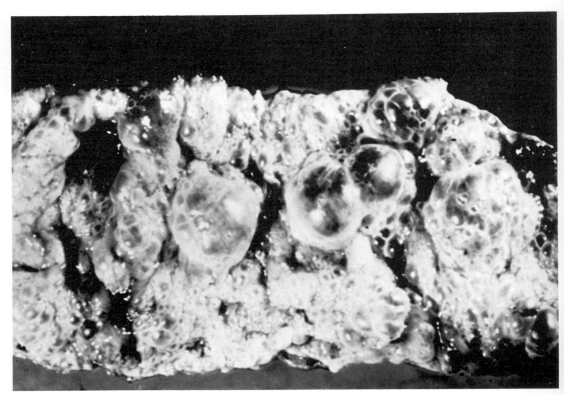

Figure 7D

may be completely reversible because of the rich collateral circulation which exists between the celiac axis, superior mesenteric, inferior mesenteric, and the middle and inferior hemorrhoidal branches of the hypogastric artery. The ultimate fate of any occlusion depends upon the collaterals, and if one or more of the major arteries mentioned are occluded, the necrosis in the infarcted area may result in fibrosis and stricture since the collateral circulation develops in time to prevent irreversible complete necrosis. When complete necrosis exists, perforation will usually occur. Arteriographic studies are of great help in making the diagnosis, although the clinical findings and roentgenographic studies such as a barium enema are often adequate to make the diagnosis.

DISCUSSION

It is difficult to prove the precise etiologic mechanisms involved in a given case of pneumatosis coli, but it is known that the most commonly associated diseases are those which cause *partial obstruction* in some part of the gastrointestinal tract, obstructive peptic ulcer disease of the pyloroduodenal

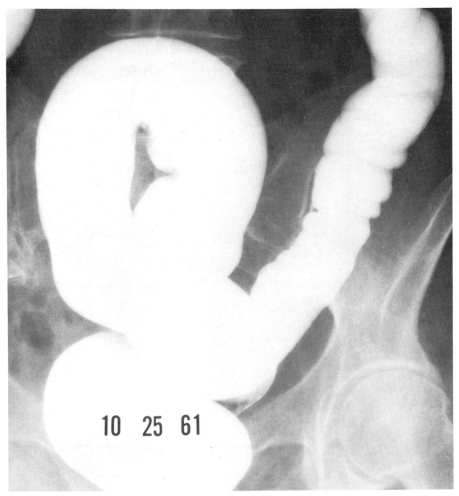

Figure 7E

region probably being the most common of these. Such obstructing lesions (see Figure 7B for diagram of this suggested mechanism) are believed to result in an increase in intraluminal pressure *proximal* to the obstructing lesions, this, in turn, apparently forcing intraluminal gas either through the intact mucosa or through small breaks in the mucosa into the wall of the bowel. From this location *proximal* to the obstruction the gas penetrates the wall to reach the subserosa from which location it can then "dissect" and extend to points far distal to the primary obstructing lesion.

Another commonly suggested mechanism is chronic obstructive pulmonary emphysema (see Figure 7C for diagram of this suggested mechanism). In this condition the alveoli are believed to rupture, with resulting passage of gas along the bronchovascular trunks into the mediastinum, from which location it dissects downward through the mediastinal tissues to reach the retroperitoneal area and thence passes between the leaves of the mesentery to reach the subserosa of the small intestine and colon.

A third cause of pneumatosis coli is trauma; e.g., that which may occur during sigmoidoscopy and the accompanying inflation of the sigmoid colon. This etiologic mechanism has been postulated in some patients in whom the condition was seen primarily on the left side of the colon.

The cause of the pneumatosis coli in the case shown here was not known because the patient had neither an obstruction in the gastrointestinal tract, nor did she have obstructive bronchopulmonary disease. She had not had a sigmoidoscopic examination prior to the barium enema. Thus, this case represents the so-called "idiopathic" form of this disease.

A photograph of a specimen (Figure 7C) from another patient with this unusual disease shows the glistening, cyst-like structures involving the entire serosal surface of the sigmoid colon.

Patients with this disease sometimes have a large pneumoperitoneum which is spectacular from a roentgenological standpoint, but is characteristically virtually asymptomatic. When first observed it may be thought due to a perforated viscus. However, once the experienced radiologist and the attending physician realize the patient is not as ill as would be expected if the large pneumoperitoneum were due to a perforated viscus, they are justified in observing the patient for several hours. If there is no change in the clinical condition of the seemingly healthy patient, a conservative approach can be adopted. The fact that such a pneumoperitoneum (often quite large) persists for months and years is evidence of a benign underlying etiological mechanism such as pneumatosis cystoides intestinalis of the small intestine or colon. Pneumatosis cystoides intestinalis of the small bowel and colon have the same etiologic mechanisms and may co-exist. The normal peritoneum can absorb about 100 cc. of air per day. Thus, when a pneumoperitoneum does not change for months or years, it is "balanced"; i.e., the amount absorbed daily by the peritoneum equals the amount which enters daily from the cysts which rupture, collapse, heal, refill, rupture again, etc.

A few cases have been reported in which this condition has disappeared spontaneously. However, documented cases are rare and illustrations of such cases are even more scarce. In the case illustrated here the sigmoid had returned to an entirely normal appearance (Figure 7E) 5 years after the original examination.

Correct roentgenological diagnosis is important when pneumatosis cystoides intestinalis is seen in the distal portion of the colon in adults, because the roentgen appearance of the barium-filled lumen of the sigmoid, at first glance, resembles the more serious conditions listed here as possible diagnoses which often may terminate with an operation.

Operation as a consequence of an erroneous diagnosis of neoplasm in cases like the one presented here has probably been carried out more frequently than indicated in the literature. However, once the diagnosis is made roentgenologically, a conservative approach is indicated and a search for the underlying chronic etiological factors (see Figures 7B and C) can be carried out. Although this condition in the colon of adults is benign, it should be emphasized that *any* intramural gas collection seen in the hollow viscera of children is usually of serious prognostic importance, as are many linear intramural gas collections in the hollow viscera of adults; i.e., they are often due to potentially lethal conditions associated with ischemic necrosis and localized or systemic infections with pathogenic gas-forming bacteria.

In summary, it is important to make the correct roentgen diagnosis of this condition because it might prevent an unnecessary operation. Furthermore, a correct diagnosis will suggest the presence of interesting etiological mechanisms which are often *remote* from the site of the roentgenologically detectable disease in the distal end of the colon. Obstructing lesions in the proximal part of the gastrointestinal tract, obstructive pulmonary emphysema and trauma coincident to sigmoidoscopy are the most frequent associated conditions which are believed to play an etiological role in the development of pneumatosis coli.

SUGGESTED READINGS

PNEUMATOSIS CYSTOIDES INTESTINALIS

1. Doub HP, Shea JJ: Pneumatosis cystoides intestinalis. JAMA *172:*1238–1242, 1960
2. Koss LG: Abdominal gas cysts (pneumatosis cystoides intestinorum hominis). Analysis with report of case and critical review of the literature. AMA Arch Pathol *53:*523–549, 1952
3. Lerner HH, Gazin AI: Pneumatosis intestinalis: its roentgenologic diagnosis. Am J Roentgenol *56:*464–469, 1946
4. Marshak RH, Blum DH, Eliasoph J: Pneumatosis including the left side of the colon. JAMA *161:*1626–1628, 1956
5. Marshak RH, Eliasoph J: Pneumatosis coli. Am J Digestive Dis, NS *1:*99–107, 1956
6. Marshak RH, Lipsay JH, Friedman AI: Pneumatosis of the colon. JAMA *148:* 1416–1417, 1952
7. Nitch CAR: Cystic pneumatosis of the intestinal tract. Brit J Surg *11:*714–735, 1924

8. Ramos AJ, Powers WE: Pneumatosis cystoides intestinalis: report of a case. Am J Roentgenol 77:678–683, 1947
9. Witkowski LJ, Pontius GV, Anderson RE: Gas cysts of the intestine. Surgery 37:959, 1955

COLITIS CYSTICA PROFUNDA
Epstein SE, Ascari WQ, Ablow RC, Seaman WB, Lattes R: Colitis cystica profunda. Am J Clin Pathol 45:186–201, 1966

CORRECT ANSWERS

Question 15-(D)
Question 16-(A)
Question 17-(E)
Question 18-(C)
Question 19-(A)

NOTES

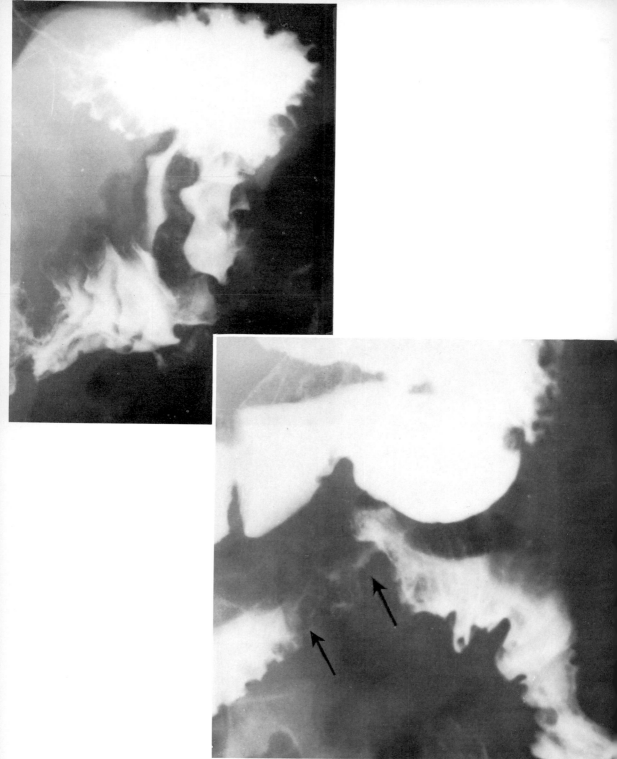

Figures 8 (top), 9 (bottom), 9-1, and 10. This 43-year-old man was examined because of persistent epigastric distress. Figure 8 is a spot roentgenogram of the stomach, Figure 9 is a spot roentgenogram of a lesion of the fourth portion of the duodenum (see *arrows*), Figure 9-1 is an upright spot roentgenogram, and Figure 10 is a postfluoroscopy roentgenogram.

Questions 20 through 24

20. Which one of the following is the *MOST* likely diagnosis?

    (A)   Crohn's disease
    (B)   Sprue
    (C)   Hodgkin's disease
    (D)   Zollinger-Ellison syndrome
    (E)   Whipple's disease

21. Which one of the following statements concerning the roentgenographic findings in Crohn's disease is *LEAST* likely?

    (A)   It may involve the stomach
    (B)   "Skip" areas are common
    (C)   There are often excessive secretions in the stomach and small intestine
    (D)   It may first present as an intestinal obstruction
    (E)   The most common site of involvement is the small bowel

22. Which one of the following combinations of small bowel roentgenographic signs is *MOST* characteristic of sprue?

    (A)   Dilatation, abnormal amount of fluid, and segmentation
    (B)   "Thumbprinting", abnormal amount of fluid, and "skip" areas
    (C)   "Thumbprinting", abnormal amount of fluid, and segmentation
    (D)   Dilatation, "string" sign, and segmentation
    (E)   Dilatation, "cobblestoning", and segmentation

23. In the Zollinger-Ellison syndrome, which one of the following is produced by non-beta islet cell tumors of the pancreas?

    (A)   Pancreatin
    (B)   Trypsin
    (C)   Secretin
    (D)   Gastrin
    (E)   Histamine

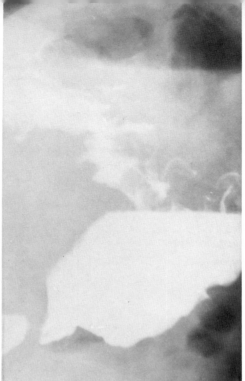

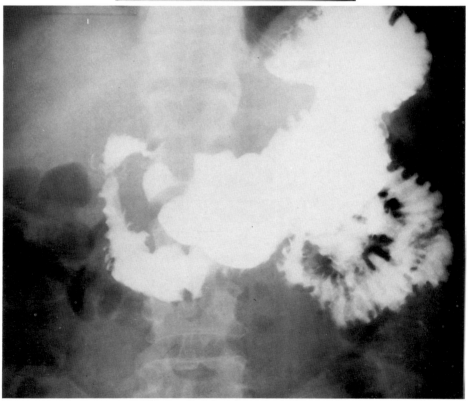

Figures 9-1 (top) and 10 (bottom)

24. Which one of the following is *MOST* typical of Whipple's disease?

   (A) Granulomatous changes in the small bowel
   (B) Periodic acid-Schiff (PAS)-positive material in the macrophages
   (C) Stenotic "skip" areas
   (D) Polypoid hyperplasia of the mucosa
   (E) Predominant ileal involvement

Discussion

QUESTION 20

The correct answer to question 20 is (D). These illustrations show several characteristic signs of the Zollinger-Ellison syndrome. Note the enlargement of the gastric mucosal folds (Figure 8), the large amount of gastric fluid (Figure 9-1), and the considerable enlargement of the mucosal folds in the jejunum (*arrows*, Figure 10C). In addition there is an abnormal narrowed area in part 3 of the duodenum (Figure 10B, *lower white arrows*) in the center of which a small barium collection indicates a shallow ulcer (Figure 10B, *upper white arrow*). Although this region is narrowed due to the edema and spasm associated with the ulcer, the mucosal folds around the ulcer are still largely intact and do not exhibit the type of destruction usually associated with carcinoma. Distal to the ulcer the jejunum is somewhat dilated and the enlarged sharply defined jejunal mucosal folds (*arrows* in Figure 10C) are highly suggestive of edema. Note also that the barium in the lumen of the somewhat dilated jejunum is diluted due to fluid (Figure 10B). When one tries to explain all of these findings on the basis of *one* etiologic mechanism, the most likely diagnosis is the Zollinger-Ellison syndrome. It is significant that there is no obstruction at the gastric outlet in this case, the pylorus (*vertical arrows* in Figures 10A and B) being normally patent, thus indicating that the large amount of gastric fluid (Figure 9-1) is probably on the basis of gastric hypersecretions rather than pyloric obstruction. Although gastric and/or duodenal ulcers are often seen in patients with the Zollinger-Ellison syndrome, none is demonstrated on these illustrations. Although the ulcers in the stomach and duodenal bulb in patients with this disease are no different in appearance from those seen in patients with ordinary peptic ulcer disease, the demonstration of a *peptic-type ulcer in the region of the ligament of Treitz*, as is seen in this case, is virtually diagnostic of the Zollinger-Ellison syndrome.

Although Crohn's disease most commonly involves the ileum, it can produce enlargement of mucosal folds in the jejunum. It can occasionally cause changes in the duodenum, but it would be extremely unusual for Crohn's disease to cause enlargement of the gastric mucosal folds as seen in this case. Furthermore, Crohn's disease could not account for the presence of excess gastric fluid unless there was an obstructing lesion in the pyloroduodenal region. No such obstruction is seen here. Thus, although it is conceivable that Crohn's disease might produce a narrowed segment in the distal part of the duodenum as shown here (Figure 9) one would not consider Crohn's disease as the diagnosis because the other findings shown here are so much against this diagnosis.

Sprue is not a tenable diagnosis because it would not be associated with marked enlargement of the gastric mucosal folds and gastric hypersecretions. Neither can the lesion in the third portion of the duodenum be explained on the basis of sprue. Although enlargement of the jejunal mucosal folds may be a relatively early finding in patients with sprue, it is more characteristic to see a diminution in the size and number of the mucosal folds. In sprue there is often some dilatation of the proximal small intestine associated with a rather mottled granular appearance of the barium owing to its mixing with abnormal amounts of fluid and other intraluminal contents, as opposed to the more "watery" type of dilution seen here. One also sees considerable moulage formation and segmentation in sprue, neither of which findings is present in the illustrations shown here

It would be somewhat unusual for Hodgkin's disease to produce enlargement of the gastric mucosal folds as seen here, although it can, admittedly, produce localized lesions which resemble the scirrhous type of gastric carcinoma. In the absence of obstruction it is also difficult to explain the excessive amount of gastric fluid seen here on the basis of Hodgkin's disease or other lymphomatous lesions of the stomach which are usually associated with a "dry" mucosa (see Figures 25 and 26, p. 130). Neither would Hodgkin's disease ordinarily cause enlargement of mucosal folds in the duodenum and jejunum, although a localized lesion could conceivably cause narrowing of the lumen as seen in the third part of the duodenum here. However, the narrowed areas produced by Hodgkin's disease are usually more tapered than the area seen here and they resemble strictures because of the fibrosis associated with this disease. The appearance of the "wet bowel" in this case is due to the large amount of gastric secretions which dilutes the barium. Such a finding would not be characteristic of Hodgkin's disease.

The radiological findings of Whipple's disease are limited almost entirely to the jejunum where it is characteristic to see a moderate degree of dilatation and enlarged mucosal folds which often appear quite irregular due to small nodules which project from the surface of the folds (see Figures 24A and B, p. 122). Whipple's disease would not be associated with the marked enlargement of the gastric mucosal folds and the excessive amount of fluid in the stomach as seen in this case. The narrowing and ulceration of the third part of the duodenum as seen here have not been reported in any part of the small intestine in Whipple's disease.

QUESTION 21

In question 21 the correct answer is (C) because the presence of excessive secretions in the stomach and small intestine is *not* a feature of Crohn's disease. However, the other listed statements concerning Crohn's disease are all true.

QUESTION 22

The correct answer to question 22 is (A). Each of the other possible answers consists of a *combination* of findings which includes at least *one* radiographic sign *not* seen in sprue; e.g., "thumbprinting", "skip" areas, "string" sign, and "cobblestoning". "Thumbprinting" usually indicates an intramural hemorrhage, whereas "skip" areas, the "string" sign, and "cobblestoning" are terms used to describe some of the common radiographic signs of Crohn's disease.

QUESTION 23

In question 23 the correct answer is (D). The pancreatic tumors which cause the Zollinger-Ellison syndrome consist of non-beta islet cells which apparently secrete *gastrin* continuously 24 hours per day. The continuous high blood level of this hormone results in a strong stimulus to the gastric parietal cells which form hydrochloric acid. The constant stimulus (see Figure 10F for the mechanism of gastrin effect on HCl secretion) to the entire parietal cell mass of the stomach is one of the factors causing large gastric mucosal folds (Figures 10A and D). Thus, the often small non-beta islet cell tumor of the pancreas can cause voluminous gastric hypersecretions and gastric hyperacidity which lead to a clinical picture of severe, often intractable, peptic ulcer disease. Although the peptic ulcerations in the Zollinger-Ellison syndrome are most common in the stomach and duodenal bulb, they are sometimes seen in unusual locations such as the esophagus, the distal duodenum (*top white arrow*, Figure 10B), and jejunum (*arrows*, Figure 10E). The patient may also have diarrhea due to the large amount of acid gastric secretions which enter and irritate the small intestine.

Questions 20 through 24 / 59

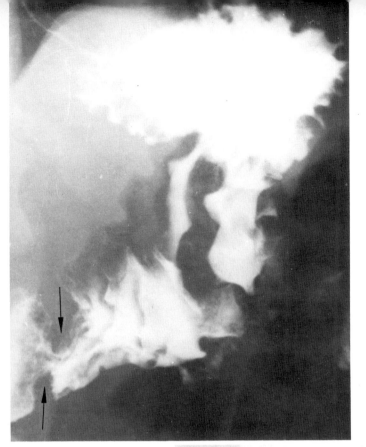

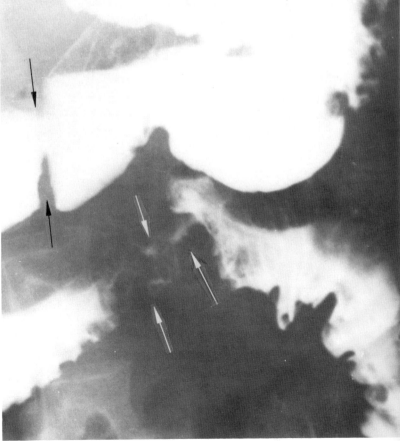

Figures 10A (top) and B (bottom)

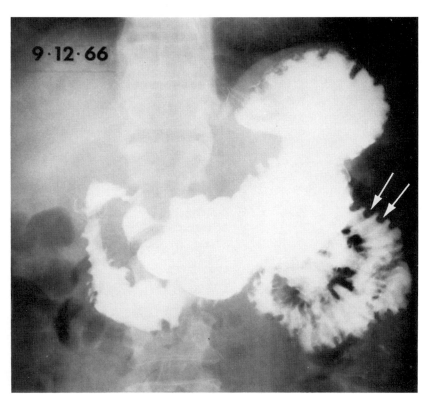

Figure 10C

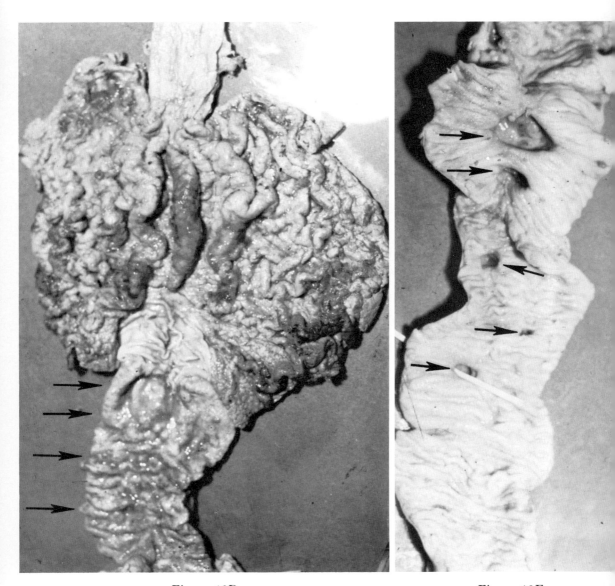

Figure 10D

Figure 10E

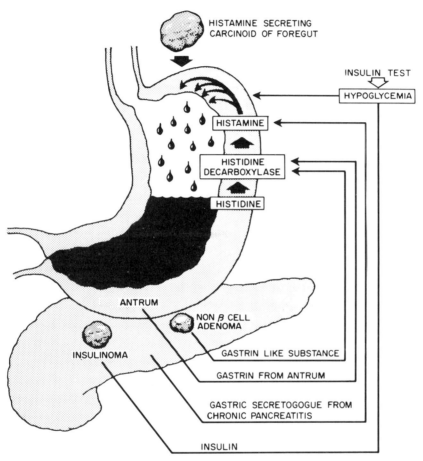

HISTAMINE SECRETING
CARCINOID OF FOREGUT

INSULIN TEST

HYPOGLYCEMIA

HISTAMINE

HISTIDINE
DECARBOXYLASE

HISTIDINE

ANTRUM

NON β CELL
ADENOMA

INSULINOMA

GASTRIN LIKE SUBSTANCE

GASTRIN FROM ANTRUM

GASTRIC SECRETOGOGUE FROM
CHRONIC PANCREATITIS

INSULIN

Figure 10F

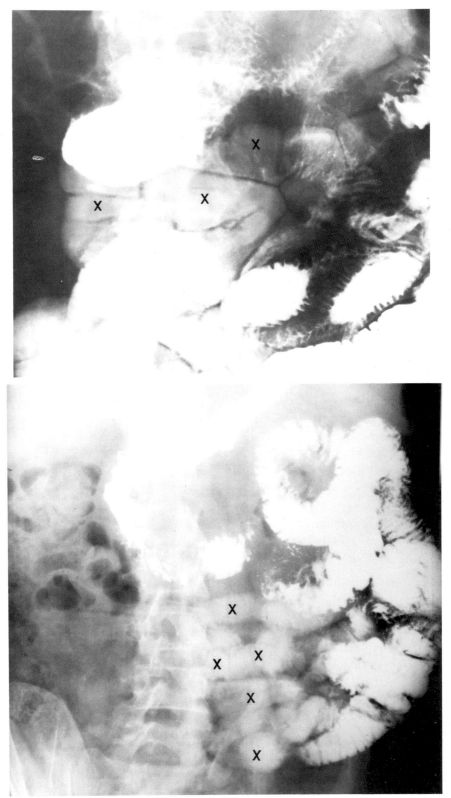

Figures 10G (top) and H (bottom)

The unusual location of the peptic ulcers seen distal to the duodenal bulb is explainable on the basis of the fact that the unusually large volume of highly-acid gastric fluid continually flows through the duodenum where the low (acid) pH cannot be sufficiently raised by the biliary and pancreatic secretions, the end result being an environment in which the pH is too low (too acid), thus leading to the production of severe inflammation and ulceration in the vulnerable distal portions of the duodenum and proximal part of the jejunum which are normally not exposed to such acid contents (see multiple ulcers in proximal jejunum in Figure 10E, *arrows*). The mucosal pattern of the more distal part of the small intestine is usually normal in the Zollinger-Ellison syndrome because the acid gastric contents which adversely affect the duodenum and jejunum become progressively diluted with normal succus entericus with a resulting rise in pH toward a more normal level as the bowel contents move distally. The excessive fluid which enters the small intestine from the stomach often results in considerable *dilution* of the barium which can often be appreciated on roentgenograms (Figures 10B, G, and H).

QUESTION 24

In question 24 the correct answer is (B) because the change most typical of Whipple's disease is the presence of periodic acid Schiff (PAS)-positive material in the macrophages in the submucosa of the jejunum (see Figures 24C and D, p. 123). In Whipple's disease there are no granulomatous changes in the jejunum, and no "skip" areas. Furthermore, the abnormal small bowel findings in Whipple's disease are *not* ordinarily seen in the ileum, but are almost always confined to the jejunum. There is no polypoid hyperplasia of the mucosa in Whipple's disease, although one may occasionally see a few scattered tiny nodules projecting from the surface of the jejunal mucosal folds (see Figures 24A, and B, *arrows*, p. 122) owing to the abnormal deposits of PAS-positive material and the dilated lymphatics in the often markedly enlarged villi, thus causing a roentgen picture which may simulate tiny mucosal "polyps".

DISCUSSION

When the stomach is full of fluid in the absence of obstructive pyloro-duodenal disease, the presence of gastric *hypersecretions* should be suspected, provided that the patient has not ingested fluid prior to the examination. However, the mere *presence* of gastric hypersecretions is not diagnostic of the Zollinger-Ellison syndrome, because there are other causes for excessive gastric secretions (Figure 10F). For instance, in chronic pancreatitis the pancreas produces a gastric secretogogue similar to, or identical to, gastrin. Gastric hypersecretion can also be produced by injecting histamine which is the basis of the augmented histamine test. It is also of interest that carcinoid tumors of the foregut (tracheobronchial tree, esophagus, and stomach) can produce large amounts of histamine which can enter the blood stream to stimulate the secretion of hydrochloric acid by the parietal cell mass of the stomach. For example, in mast cell leukemia ("mastocytosis") the large population of mast cells can produce excessive amounts of endogenous histamine (as well as serotonin and heparin) with resultant gastric hypersecretions. Insulin produces hypoglycemia which, in turn, can produce vagal stimulation leading to gastric hypersecretion. Thus, an insulin-secreting islet cell tumor of the pancreas may sometimes be associated with gastric hypersecretion.

The gross specimen of the resected stomach (Figure 10D) shows enormous enlargement of the mucosal folds (center of specimen), much of which is due to the hyperplasia of the parietal cell mass, although there is usually some edema, too. The esophagus (Figure 10D, *pale structure at top of figure*) was normal in this case, although ulcers of the lower esophagus do occasionally occur in this disease. Note the absence of ulcer in the duodenum (Figure 10D, *arrows, lower part of the figure*), although the enlarged duodenal edematous folds indicate duodenitis. Figure 10E is the autopsy specimen of the proximal jejunum of another patient who died as a result of a perforated jejunal ulcer (see *toothpick* inserted through the perforation in Figure 10E). Note that there are a total of five jejunal ulcers (*arrows*, Figure 10E).

It should be emphasized that the gastrointestinal symptoms of the Zollinger-Ellison syndrome almost always lead to one or more roentgen examinations. Consequently, the radiologist can be the first to make, or at least strongly suggest, the diagnosis if he is cognizant of the significance of the *combination* of the roentgen findings shown here. These characteristic findings are (1) gastric hypersecretions, (2) large mucosal folds in the stomach, duodenum, and proximal jejunum, (3) peptic ulcers occurring around the region of the ligament of Treitz, and (4) dilution of the barium suspension in the small intestine. Dilution of the barium in the small intestine was not particularly noticeable on the illustrations shown to you, although the majority of the typical roentgen findings are seen in this case. However, on illustrations (Figures 10G and H) of roentgenograms of two other patients with the Zollinger-Ellison syndrome, note the gray "watery" appearance of the barium in several loops ("x" in Figures 10G and H) as compared to the more normal density of the barium in the more proximal loops. Since the ingested barium suspension settles to the distal end of the fluid-filled stomach when the patient is in the erect or prone position, it often enters the duodenum in a relatively undiluted state (normal density) and seems to "chase", but does not mix well with, the excessive fluid already in the small intestine. Thus, the abnormal amount of fluid in the small bowel in patients with the Zollinger-Ellison syndrome may be indicated by barely enough mixing to permit some opacification of the otherwise invisible fluid-filled loops of bowel at the distal end of the barium column.

This case was presented in order to illustrate and correlate the roentgen findings in the Zollinger-Ellison syndrome and to emphasize the importance of trying to explain *all* of the roentgen findings in the stomach, duodenum, and jejunum on the basis of *one* disease. Your ability to suggest this important diagnosis will be improved by understanding the underlying pathophysiological mechanisms responsible for the production of these signs. In this patient a benign non-beta islet cell adenoma of the pancreas only *1 cm. in diameter* produced these severe changes! It is important to remember that the prognosis for *survival* of the patient is usually directly related to the length of time required to make the diagnosis and perform the required *total gastrectomy*. About 50 per cent of these neoplasms are malignant, and the gastrin produced by the metastases (usually in the liver) will *continue* to stimulate the parietal cell mass in any gastric remnant present after the usual peptic ulcer operations, *even though the primary tumor of the pancreas has been removed, or though a total pancreatectomy has been performed*. Thus, it is generally believed desirable to remove the entire target organ (parietal cell mass of the stomach) by doing a *total gastrectomy*. In undiagnosed cases death is usually the result of the complications of rapidly recurring fulminating peptic ulcer disease after repeated ordinary peptic ulcer operations.

SUGGESTED READINGS

ZOLLINGER-ELLISON SYNDROME

1. Amberg JR, Ellison EH, Wilson SD, Zboralske FF: Roentgenographic observations in the Zollinger-Ellison syndrome. JAMA *190:*185–187, 1964
2. Christoforidis AJ, Nelson SW: Radiological manifestations of ulcerogenic tumors of the pancreas: the Zollinger-Ellison syndrome. JAMA *198:*511–516, 1966
3. Ellison EH, Wilson SD: The Zollinger-Ellison syndrome: re-appraisal and evaluation of 260 registered cases. Ann Surg *160:*512–528, 1964
4. Missakian MM, Carlson HC, Huizenga KA: Roentgenographic findings in Zollinger-Ellison syndrome. Am J Roentgenol *94:*429–437, 1965
5. Nelson SW, Christoforidis AJ: Roentgenologic features of the Zollinger-Ellison syndrome—ulcerogenic tumor of the pancreas. Semin in Roentgenol *3:* 254–265, 1968
6. Zboralski FF, Amberg JR: Detection of the Zollinger-Ellison syndrome: the radiologist's responsibility. Am J Roentgenol *104:*529–543, 1968

SPRUE

Marshak RH, Lindner AE: *Radiology of the Small Intestine*, pp 11–29. WB Saunders Co, Philadelphia, 1970

HODGKIN'S DISEASE

Marshak RH, Lindner AE: *Radiology of the Small Intestine*, pp 384–389. WB Saunders Co, Philadelphia, 1970

WHIPPLE'S DISEASE

1. Clement AR, Marshak RH: Whipple's disease: roentgen features and differential diagnosis. Radiol Clin North Am 7:105–110, 1969
2. Marshak RH, Lindner AE: *Radiology of the Small Intestine*, pp 40–50. WB Saunders Co, Philadelphia, 1970
3. Martel W, Hodges FJ: The small intestine in Whipple's disease. Am J Roentgenol 81:623–636, 1959
4. Rice RP, Roufail W, Reeves RJ: The roentgen diagnosis of Whipple's disease (intestinal lipodystrophy), with emphasis on improvement following antibiotic therapy. Radiology 88:295–301, 1967
5. Schatzki SC: Whipple's disease. Roentgenologic findings, including those of eight-year remissions. Radiology 75:908–913, 1960
6. Triano GJ: Further roentgen observations on the small intestine in Whipple's disease. Am J Roentgenol 87:717–720, 1962

CORRECT ANSWERS

Question 20-(D)
Question 21-(C)
Question 22-(A)
Question 23-(D)
Question 24-(B)

NOTES

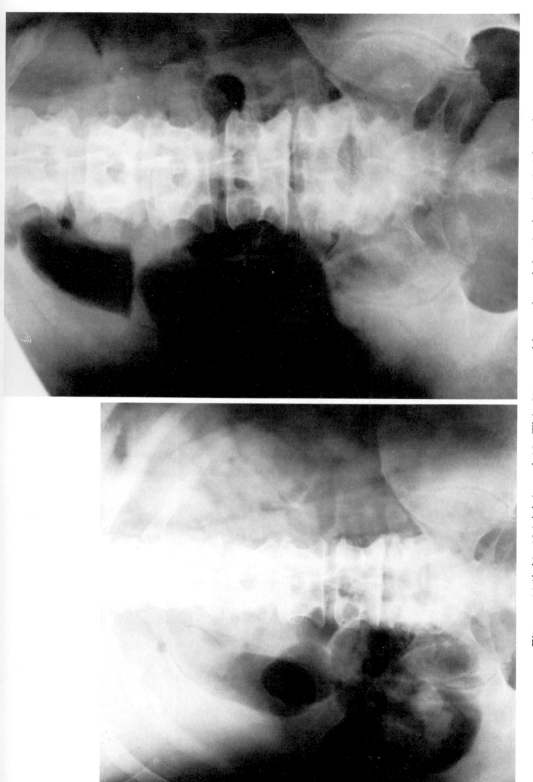

Figures 11 (left), 12 (right), and 13. This 65-year-old man has abdominal pain of 10 hours' duration. Roentgenograms of the abdomen were taken with the patient in the supine (Figure 11), upright (Figure 12), and upright oblique (Figure 13) positions.

Questions 25 through 29

25. Which one of the following is the *MOST* likely diagnosis?

    (A) Pancreatitis
    (B) Emphysematous cholecystitis
    (C) Duodenal obstruction
    (D) Appendicitis
    (E) Obstruction of the transverse colon

26. Which one of the following conditions is *LEAST* likely to produce pancreatitis?

    (A) Diabetes
    (B) Alcoholism
    (C) Gallstones
    (D) Abdominal surgery
    (E) Trauma

27. Emphysematous cholecystitis is associated *MOST* frequently with which one of the following?

    (A) Common duct stricture
    (B) Gallstones
    (C) Diabetes
    (D) Adenomyomatosis
    (E) Ascending cholangitis

28. In a patient with right lower quadrant pain, the single roentgenographic finding which is *MOST* suggestive of appendicitis is

    (A) failure to fill the appendix on a barium enema
    (B) air-fluid levels in the right lower quadrant
    (C) an oval calcification in the right lower quadrant
    (D) loss of the right psoas shadow
    (E) loss of the properitoneal fat line

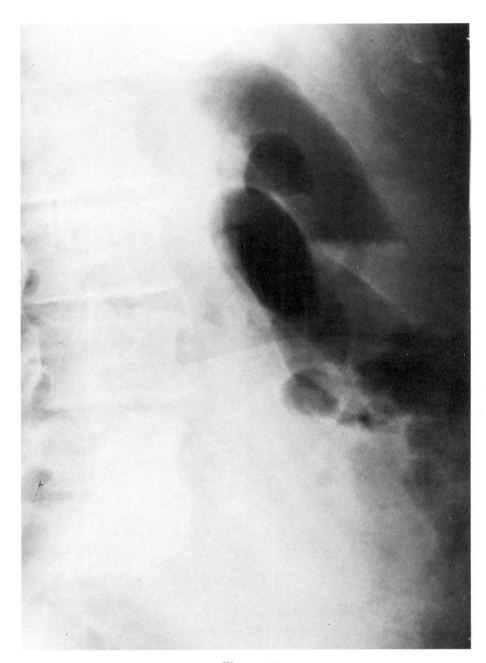

Figure 13

29. Dilatation of the transverse colon is *LEAST* commonly produced by which one of the following?

   (A)   Carcinoma of the colon
   (B)   Pancreatitis
   (C)   Acute cholecystitis
   (D)   Amebiasis
   (E)   Ileocolic intussusception

Discussion

QUESTION 25

Figures 11, 12, and 13 demonstrate an air-filled structure within the right upper quadrant which shows an air-fluid level on the upright projection. In the recumbent view (Figure 11), gas can be seen within the wall of this structure. Several small bowel loops in the same area are dilated.

The correct answer, therefore, **to question 25 is "emphysematous cholecystitis" (B),** as these are the roentgen manifestations of this condition. The dilated small bowel loops represent localized ileus in response to the adjacent inflammatory reaction of the gallbladder.

Your first impression might be a dilated duodenum because of the location of the gas-filled gallbladder. However, the lack of evidence of gastric obstruction or a dilated duodenal bulb is against this diagnosis.

Although pancreatitis and appendicitis may be associated with localized dilatation of small bowel loops ("sentinel loops"), the identification of the gas-filled gallbladder excludes these diagnoses.

QUESTION 26

In question 26, alcoholism, gallstones, abdominal surgery, and trauma are all frequently associated with or causes of pancreatitis. Although severe pancreatitis may result in the development of diabetes, diabetes itself is not a cause of pancreatitis. Therefore, **your answer to question 26 should be (A).**

The greatest incidence of emphysematous cholecystitis is in the fourth and fifth decades and appears to be more common in men than in women. There is no classical clinical picture since the findings in this disease are in no way different from cholecystitis without gas formation. Although there appears to be a higher incidence of diabetes mellitus in patients with chole-cystitis (about 25 per cent), the hallmark and basic cause of emphysema-tous cholecystitis is almost invariably *obstruction of the cystic duct*, most often by stones. This has also been shown experimentally. *Escherichia coli*, Staphylococcus, Streptococcus, and Clostridia have all been incriminated bacteria. These microorganisms may be associated with the routine forms of cholecystitis and may also be found in the bile of apparently healthy gall-bladders. It is therefore believed that it is the cystic duct obstruction that changes the physiology of the gallbladder (stasis, ischemia, etc.), permit-ting development of emphysematous cholecystitis. However, we have ob-served emphysematous cholecystitis and biliary air (Figure 13A, *arrow*) de-veloping in a patient subsequent to arteriography even though a gallbladder series 24 hours earlier had demonstrated a normal gallbladder without calculi. Embolization of the cystic artery, although not proved in our post-arteriography case, appears to have been the probable cause of the gangrene because pathologic evaluation revealed thrombosis of all branches of the cystic artery and necrosis of the gallbladder wall.

The correct answer to question 27 is (B) because "gallstones" is the only listed condition associated with cystic duct obstruction.

All of the conditions listed in question 28 have been described with acute appendicitis. However, the presence of an **oval calcification within the right lower quadrant (C)** in a patient with abdominal pain is essentially diagnostic of appendicitis secondary to an appendicolith. Failure to fill the appendix on a barium enema is meaningless. Air-fluid levels in the right lower quadrant, loss of the right psoas shadow, and loss of the properitoneal fat line are only suggestive of appendicitis as they can be seen in healthy patients or with other inflammatory conditions.

About 10 per cent of all patients with acute appendicitis have demon-strable fecaliths radiographically. Their presence is of extreme importance, since the incidence of gangrene and perforation is quite high, exceeding 90 per cent in some series.

In the opinion of most surgeons, the demonstration of a calculus in this area is indication for appendectomy. Most appendiceal calculi are roughly 1 cm. in diameter, oval, and frequently laminated. It must be pointed out

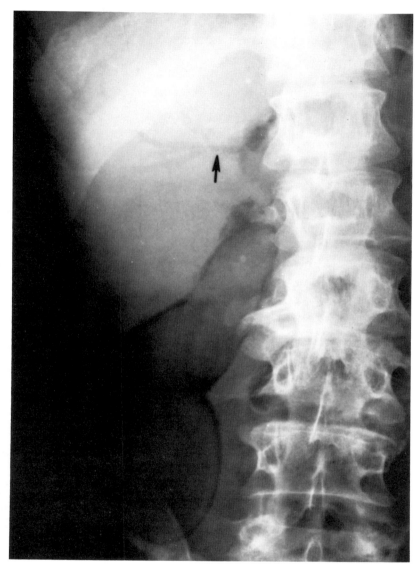

Figure 13A

that the identification of calculi within the right upper quadrant or left lower quadrant must also raise the question of appendicitis. The differential diagnosis must, of course, include calculus within a Meckel's diverticulum and, in the older age group, calculus within a colonic diverticulum.

QUESTION 29

In question 29 all of the lesions described may be associated with dilatation of the transverse colon except **ileocolic intussusception (E),** which is, therefore, the correct answer.

Dilatation of the transverse colon with pancreatitis or acute cholecystitis is usually due to a localized ileus ("sentinel" loop) resulting from an adjacent inflammatory reaction.

Toxic dilatation of the colon is more frequently seen in ulcerative colitis but can be seen in amebiasis. Carcinoma of the colon, which occurs most commonly on the left side, generally causes dilatation proximally including the transverse colon.

SUGGESTED READINGS

1. Donner MW, Weiner S: Diagnostic evaluation of abdominal calcifications in acute abdominal disorders. Radiol Clin North Am 2:145–159, 1964
2. Evans JA: Biliary tract problems in the aged. Radiol Clin North Am 3:305–319, 1965
3. Felson B, Bernhard CM: The roentgenologic diagnosis of appendiceal calculi. Radiology 49:178–191, 1947
4. Frimann-Dahl J: Roentgen Examinations in Acute Abdominal Diseases. Charles C Thomas, Springfield, Ill, 1960
5. Grainger K: Acute emphysematous cholecystitis: report of a case. Clin Radiol 12:66–69, 1961
6. Nelson SW: Extraluminal gas collections due to diseases of the gastrointestinal tract. Am J Roentgenol 115:225–248, 1972
7. Schowengerdt CG, Wiot JF: Emphysematous cholecystitis following aortography. Am Surgeon 35:274–277, 1972

CORRECT ANSWERS

Question 25-(B)
Question 26-(A)
Question 27-(B)
Question 28-(C)
Question 29-(E)

NOTES

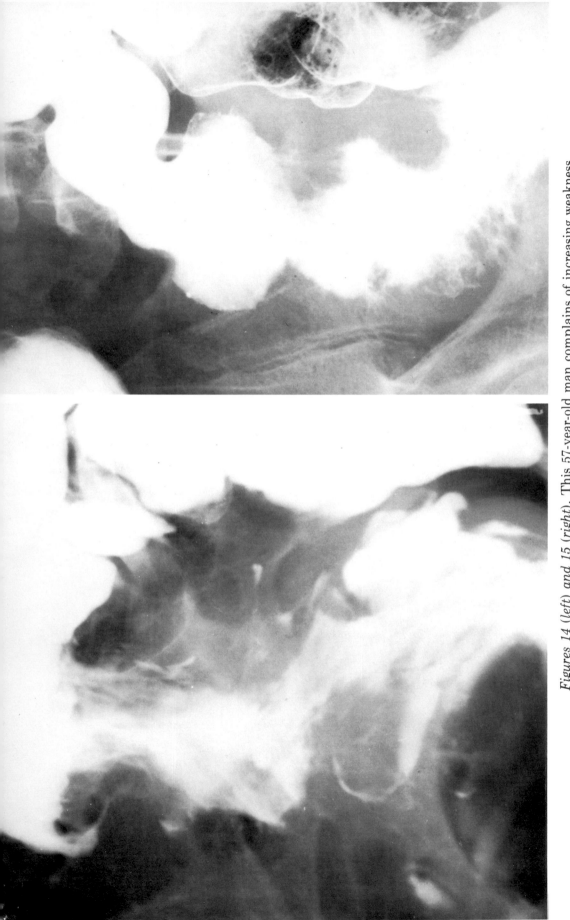

Figures 14 (left) and 15 (right). This 57-year-old man complains of increasing weakness and easy fatigability. Figure 14 is a roentgenogram of the barium-filled rectum and Figure 15 is a postevacuation view.

Questions 30 through 35

30. Which one of the following is the *MOST* likely diagnosis?

    (A) Carcinoma
    (B) Villous adenoma
    (C) Lymphosarcoma
    (D) Hemangioma
    (E) Metastasis

For each of the numbered clinical disorders listed below (Questions 31–34), select the *one* lettered characteristic (A,B,C,D,E) that is *MOST* closely associated with it. Each lettered characteristic may be selected once, more than once, or not at all.

    (A) Frequent calcification
    (B) Angulation of loops
    (C) Softness and pliability
    (D) Marked mesenteric involvement
    (E) Often circumferential

31. Carcinoma

32. Villous adenoma

33. Lymphosarcoma

34. Metastasis

35. Which one of the following statements concerning villous adenomas is *MOST* likely?

    (A) They are firm in consistency
    (B) They are most common in the cecum
    (C) They are often pedunculated
    (D) They may be associated with serum electrolyte imbalance
    (E) They have a low potential for malignancy

Discussion

QUESTION 30

The correct answer to question 30 is (B). The view of the filled rectum (Figure 14) shows a huge bulky mass which, at first glance, looks like an annular carcinoma encircling the entire circumference of the rectum. The proximal (upper) margin of the lesion appears to have a "shelf" or overhanging mushroom-shaped edge and in the main portion of the mass there are a few streaks of barium extending from the lumen into the mass (Figure 15A, *arrows*). However, note the interesting change in appearance of the mass as seen on the postevacuation view (Figure 15). The mass now looks much smaller, and it has a striking striated "brush-like" margin which differs from the appearance of the filled view which shows only a few larger streaks of barium extending into the mass (Figure 15A, *arrows*). Close inspection of the postevacuation view shows multiple tiny projections (Figure 15B, *arrows*) of barium extending into the lesion. Note the fine "lace-like" pattern of the barium (Figure 15B, in the area indicated by the *lower arrow*).

Could this be a carcinoma? An annular carcinoma of the rectum is rarely as large as the tumor seen here. Furthermore, a carcinoma does not have the innumerable fine streaks of barium extending into it and would thus not exhibit the striated "brush-like" border seen here. An annular carcinoma would also be too rigid to allow for the remarkable change in the caliber of the lumen seen here. Thus, carcinoma is not a very likely possibility in this case.

Lymphosarcomas can be as large as the tumor seen here and they do sometimes occur in the rectum. However, they are not characterized by a striated "brush-like" border or a change in size as is seen in the lesion illustrated here. Furthermore, primary lymphosarcomas of the rectum usually have a nodular or polypoid surface, whereas extrinsic lymphosarcoma which invade by contiguity usually do not produce complete annular involvement of the rectum, but tend to indent it from one or more aspects.

Hemangiomas sometimes occur in the rectum, and they often contain the characteristic multiple round or oval-shaped calcified phleboliths which, if present, almost always give a good clue to the correct diagnosis. Furthermore, their surfaces are smooth and do not produce the lace-like pattern seen in this case.

Intraperitoneal "drop" metastases to the pelvis from other abdominal tumors (e.g., stomach) do not ordinarily produce annular lesions of the rectum, but would tend to involve the anterior wall which is covered by peri-

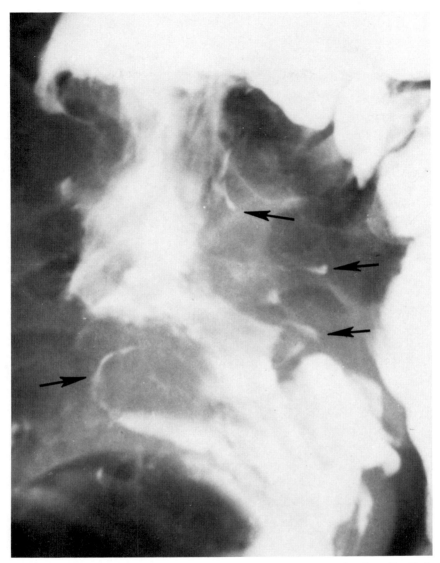

Figure 15A. From Frye TF: Villous adenoma of the sigmoid colon. Radiology *73:*71–75, 1959 (with permission of the author and publisher).

toneum. However, carcinoma of the prostate or uterine cervix can sometimes produce narrowing and rigidity of the rectum. Such rigid lesions would have an unchanging appearance on roentgenograms, in contrast to the soft consistency of the lesion seen here, as manifested by a considerable change in size after evacuation. Indeed, if the circumferential lesion seen here were due to metastatic disease, it would very likely be associated with a frozen pelvis, both clinically and roentgenologically.

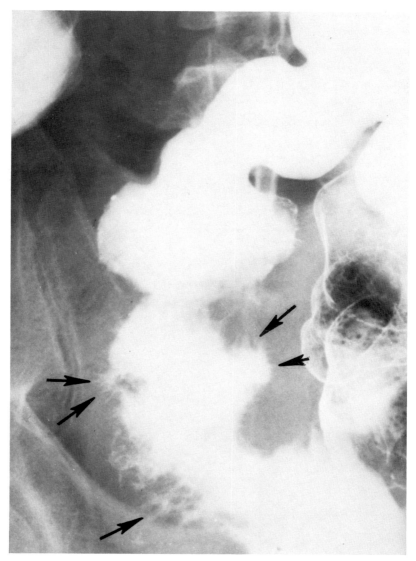

Figure 15B. From Frye TF: Villous adenoma of the sigmoid colon. Radiology 73:71–75, 1959 (with permission of the author and publisher).

QUESTION 31

The correct answer to question 31 is (E) because the word "circumferential" refers to the annular shape which is so characteristic of many carcinomas.

QUESTION 32

The correct answer to question 32 is (C) because softness and pliability are characteristics *most* closely associated with villous adenomas.

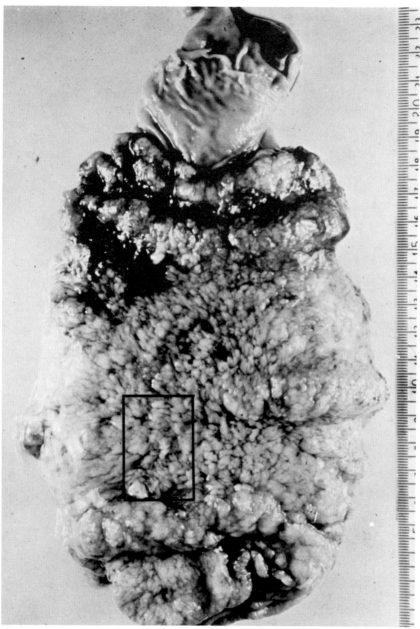

Figure 15C. From Frye TF: Villous adenoma of the sigmoid colon. Radiology 73:71–75, 1959 (with permission of the author and publisher).

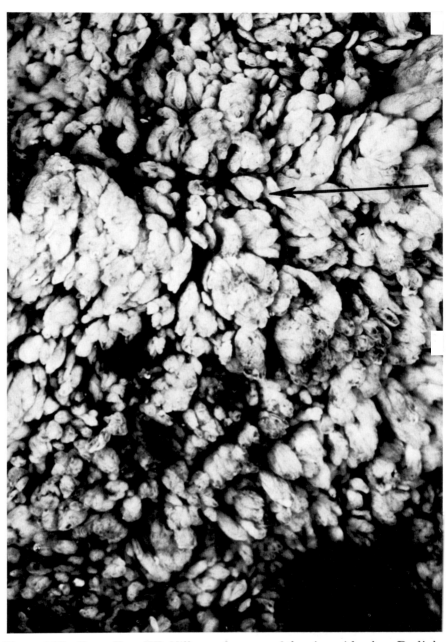

Figure 15D. From Frye TF: Villous adenoma of the sigmoid colon. Radiology 73:71–75, 1959 (with permission of the author and publisher).

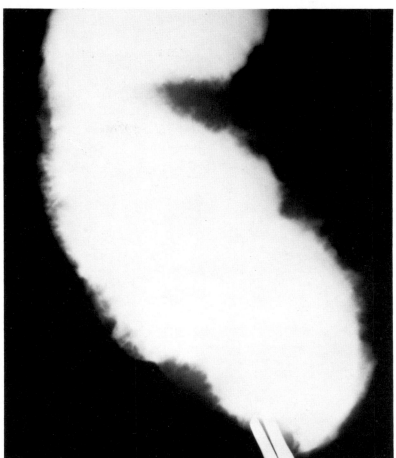

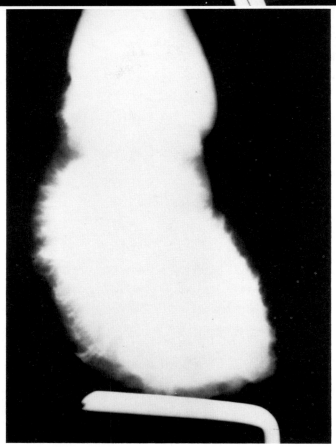

Figures 15E (top) and F (bottom)

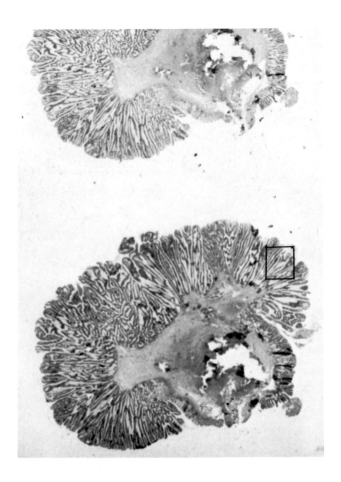

QUESTION 33

The correct answer to question 33 is (D), the mesenteric involvement probably being related to the fact that many lymphosarcomas originate in the lymph nodes in the mesentery and invade the mesenteric side of the bowel wall by contiguity.

QUESTION 34

Peritoneal metastases frequently produce angulation and kinking of small bowel loops due to the fact that a metastatic lesion between two adjacent loops causes them to adhere to one another. Thus, **the correct answer to question 34 is (B).**

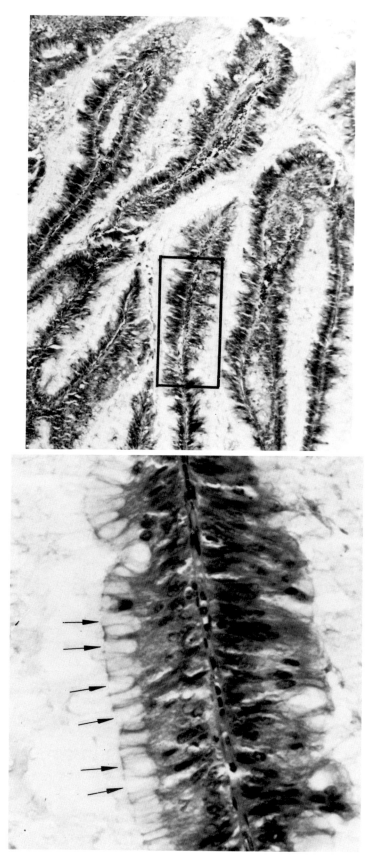

Figures 15H (top) and I (bottom)

QUESTION 35

The correct answer to question 35 is (D) and the cause of this tendency to produce serum electrolyte imbalance will be mentioned later in the discussion. None of the other listed possible answers is true of villous adenomas.

DISCUSSION

The roentgen findings shown here are characteristic for a villous adenoma and can easily be explained on the basis of the gross and microscopic characteristics shown on the photographs of the lesion (Figures 15C, D, E, and F) which were made after an anterior resection of the lesion. In order to photograph the characteristic surface appearance of a villous adenoma the tube-like specimen has been pulled "inside out" (Figure 15C) as one would a stocking, thus exposing the everted surface of the tumor which involves the entire circumference of the specimen. It is possible to pull this specimen "inside out" because the soft tumor is limited entirely to the mucosa, thus leaving the muscular wall of the rectosigmoid normal in pliability. Note the shaggy surface of the tumor due to the innumerable mucosal projections or "fronds" which have the same soft consistency as normal mucosa. These innumerable soft "fronds" cause the surface of this bulky tumor to have a velvety appearance and a soft mushy texture due to the large amount of mucus between the "fronds." The close-up view of the "fronds" (Figure 15D is an enlargement of the rectangular area in Figure 15C) was made possible by photographing the lesion through clear saline in which the specimen was immersed so as to allow the innumerably floating polyp-like "fronds" to be more clearly visible as the saline separated them by flowing between them. These gross characteristics can thus be correlated with the appearance of the barium enema illustrations shown here. Two roentgenograms of the resected specimen made at right angles to each other (Figures 15E and F) provided a more spectacular correlation. The distal end of the specimen was occluded with a clamp after which a water-soluble iodinated medium was introduced into the lumen. It was then radiographed in the erect position to permit gravity to aid in the filling of the spaces between the "fronds", thus producing a striking demonstration of the striated "brush-like" surface which we saw clearly, but less spectacularly, on the postevacuation view (Figure 5B, *arrows*). This "brush-like" appearance of the surface is a characteristic roentgen finding of this interesting lesion.

If one of the tiny polyp-like "fronds" (*arrow* in Figure 15D) is examined under low power (Figure 15G), it is indeed seen to resemble a tiny polyp. The mucosal surface of each "frond" is thrown into hundreds of undulating crowded villi, which arrangement creates an enormous mucosal surface area because of the large number of "fronds" (Figures 15C and D). A high-power view of a few of these villi (Figure 15H, which corresponds to the small square area in Figure 15G) shows that their surface is covered by a layer of columnar epithelium. A more magnified view of *one* of the villi (Figure 15I, which corresponds to the small rectangular area in Figure 15H) shows that the majority of the epithelial cells are goblet cells which are discharging mucus into the lumen (*arrows* in Figure 15I). The great number of goblet cells and the large mucosal surface area of a villous adenoma explain the secretion of such copious amounts of thick mucus by these tumors. The large amount of mucus which accumulates between the "fronds" helps explain the fact that relatively little barium could enter these spaces at the beginning of the barium enema (Figure 14), at which time the mucus in the bowel lumen also caused a somewhat blurred stringy appearance of the intraluminal barium. However, the postevacuation film (Figure 15) was made after several rectal contractions had caused the mucus to be squeezed out of these spaces between the "fronds" so that residual barium could enter them when the rectum relaxed again, thus producing the striated "brush-like" appearance on the postevacuation roentgenogram. The squeezing of large amounts of mucus out of the interstices of such a tumor by the rectal contractions also explains why this type of tumor often appears to decrease in size after evacuation.

The enormous amount of mucus lost by rectum in a patient with such a large villous adenoma may lead to a dangerous depletion of serum electrolytes and proteins. While in the hospital prior to his operation, this patient passed up to 2000 cc. of mucus per day by rectum, each liter of which contained 114 meq. of sodium, 19 meq. of potassium, and 120 meq. of chlorides! Fluid and electrolyte replacement resulted in prompt disappearance of his weakness and easy fatiguability, and the return of his serum electrolyte values to normal. The patient made an uneventful recovery after the tumor was resected.

It should be noted that the profuse discharge of the large amounts of mucus produced by the tumor may sometimes lead to an erroneous diagnosis of "mucus colitis". The large amount of mucus produced by the tumor can also cause considerable tenesmus and it is characteristic that the mucus which accumulated in the region of the tumor is passed *separately* from the stool; i.e., either before or after.

Villous adenomas of the colon are benign tumors, the typical radiological appearance of which was first described by Frye in 1959. These tumors are encountered primarily in late life, the average age of incidence being in the middle of the sixth decade. There is no apparent familial or sexual predilection. They usually occur as single tumors and are said to comprise about 2 per cent of all tumors of the colon and rectum. They may occur in association with additional benign or malignant neoplasms elsewhere in the colon. The only other benign epithelial tumor of the colonic mucosa is the adenomatous polyp which is a compact, spheroid, pedunculated or sessile lesion in contrast to the soft mushy villous adenoma which may vary in size from several centimeters to masses of enormous size which often completely encircle the bowel, as illustrated in this case. Although villous adenomas usually do not involve the deeper layers of the rectal wall, in approximately 50 per cent of the cases the tumors have a strong tendency toward invasion and malignant transformation. When this occurs the lesion becomes an invasive carcinoma. Some benign villous adenomas have a tendency toward recurrence after local removal, and wide excision is thus desirable in all cases.

Rectal bleeding is sometimes associated with these tumors if there is erosion of the mucosa, although it was not present in the cases shown here. Other symptoms caused by such large tumors of the rectum include a sensation of incomplete evacuation and occasional protrusion of a part of the soft bulky tumor through the anus if the lesion happens to be located in the distal part of the rectum.

In summary, when the barium enema roentgenograms show a large soft intraluminal tumor of the rectum, particularly if it involves the entire circumference, and if innumerable small streaks of barium extend into the mass of the tumor, one should think first of a villous adenoma. The diagnosis is almost certain when such a tumor appears to become smaller after evacuation, at which time the striated "brush-like" border is much better seen than on the filled views. Villous adenomas encountered in other parts of the gastrointestinal tract do not usually become as large and bulky as those which occur in the rectum, but they often have the same characteristic roentgenological findings.

SUGGESTED READINGS

VILLOUS ADENOMA

1. Fitzgerald MG: Extreme fluid and electrolyte loss due to villous papilloma of the rectum. Brit Med J *1*:831–832, 1955
2. Frye TR: Villous adenoma of the sigmoid colon. Radiology *73*:71–75, 1959
3. Henshall GK: Villous tumors of the large bowel and presentation of an unusual case. Am J Roentgenol *84*:1105–1113, 1960
4. Ryan JE: Villous tumors of the rectum below the peritoneal reflection. Am J Surg *86*:535–538, 1953

5. Wheat MW Jr, Ackerman LV: Villous adenomas of the large intestine: clinico-pathologic evaluation of 50 cases of villous adenomas with emphasis on treatment. Ann Surg *147:*476–487, 1958
6. Wolf BS: Roentgen diagnosis of villous tumors of the colon. Am J Roentgenol *84:*1093–1104, 1960

METASTASES

1. Salik JO: Extrarectal tumors caused by silent carcinomas of the stomach and pancreas. JAMA *175:*457–462, 1961
2. Zboralske FF, Bessolo RJ: Metastatic carcinoma to the mesentery and gut. Radiology *88:*302–310, 1967

LYMPHOSARCOMA

Woodruff JH Jr, Skorneck AB: Malignant lymphoma of the colon and rectum. Roentgen diagnosis. California Med *96:*181–183, 1962

CORRECT ANSWERS

Question 30-(B)
Question 31-(E)
Question 32-(C)
Question 33-(D)
Question 34-(B)
Question 35-(D)

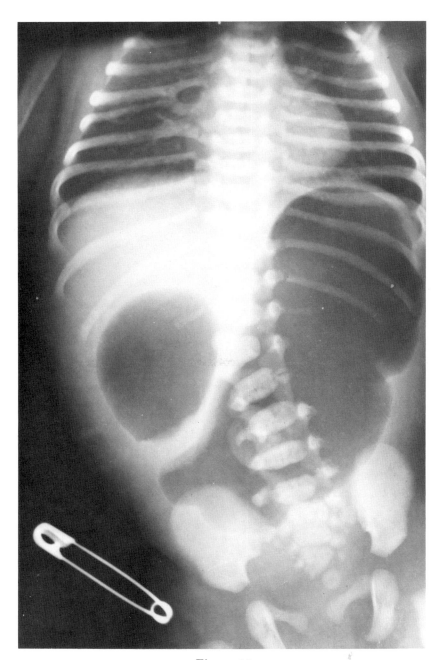

Figure 16

Figures 16 and 17. This 3-day-old girl has had persistent vomiting since birth. Roentgenograms of the abdomen were taken with the patient in the supine (Figure 16) and upright (Figure 17) positions.

Questions 36 through 40

36. Which one of the following is the *MOST* likely diagnosis on the basis of the roentgenographic findings?

    (A) Annular pancreas
    (B) Duodenal atresia
    (C) **Midgut volvulus**
    (D) Duodenal band
    (E) Communicating duplication

37. Duodenal atresia is *MOST* commonly associated with which one of the following conditions?

    (A) Mongolism
    (B) Prematurity
    (C) Maternal diabetes
    (D) Meconium ileus
    (E) None of the above

38. Which one of the following statements concerning congenital duodenal bands is *MOST* likely?

    (A) They usually obstruct the first portion of the duodenum
    (B) They usually produce complete obstructions
    (C) They are not usually associated with malrotation
    (D) **They are often seen in patients with midgut volvulus**
    (E) They are a common cause of meconium ileus

39. Which one of the following statements concerning midgut volvulus is *INCORRECT*?

    (A) It is characterized by obstruction of the third part of the duodenum
    (B) It characteristically persists until corrected surgically
    (C) It occurs in both infants and adults
    (D) The cecum usually is high in the left upper abdomen
    (E) It is often associated with obstructing peritoneal bands

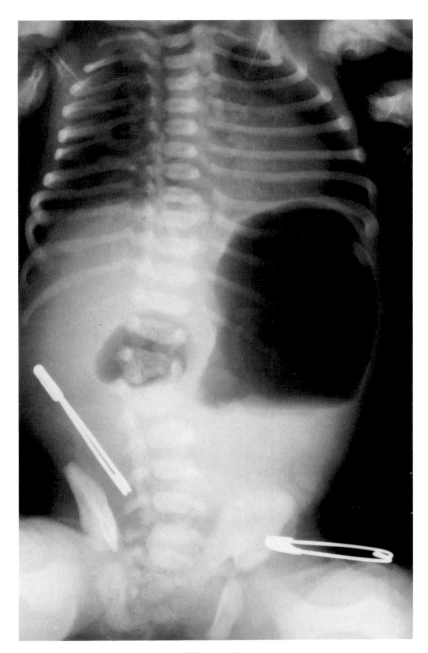

Figure 17

40. Which one of the following statements concerning annular pancreas is *INCORRECT?*

(A) It is discovered more frequently in infants than in adults
(B) It usually affects the second (descending) portion of the duodenum
(C) It most commonly causes a partial obstruction
(D) The usual roentgenographic manifestation is an indentation of the outer (convex) portion of the duodenum
(E) Peptic ulcer is often an associated complication

Discussion

QUESTION 36

The correct answer to question 36 is (B). In this condition there is atresia of the duodenum distal to the duodenal bulb, and in about 80 per cent of the cases the atretic segment is located distal to the ampulla of Vater. Duodenal atresia is the most common cause of congenital obstruction of the duodenum, and since the obstruction is always *complete* in duodenal atresia, there is no evidence of gas distal to the proximal part of the duodenum (the smallest "bubble" in Figures 16 and 17). Thus, the presence of the characteristic "double bubble" during the first few days of the infant's life, particularly when there is no roentgenographic evidence of gas distal to the distended duodenum, makes the diagnosis of duodenal atresia by far the most likely possibility.

The vast majority of patients with duodenal atresia have the onset of their symptoms within 24 hours following birth. It is also important to remember that in duodenal atresia the obstruction is so *high* in the gastrointestinal tract that the associated frequent vomiting and inability to retain fluids and electrolytes can cause the infant's condition to deteriorate rapidly unless a duodenoduodenostomy or a duodenojejunostomy is performed promptly. Therefore, an early diagnosis is not only important, but also possible in the vast majority of cases because of the presence of the so-called "double bubble" sign in an infant with symptoms of high obstruction. The largest "bubble" on the left side of the abdomen is the gas in the distended stomach, whereas the gas in the considerably distended first portion of the duodenum forms the smaller "bubble" on the right. Since duodenal atresia results from *failure of recanalization* of the duodenum between the sixth and eleventh weeks of fetal life, the duodenum proximal to the atretic segment has a long time in which to become dilated before birth. Conversely, the duodenal obstructions caused by acquired stenosis, peritoneal bands or volvulus do not usually result in as much dilatation of the duodenal bulb as is true in atresia. This is because the obstructions due to the former conditions apparently develop at a much later period of intrauterine life, and are often incomplete, thus often precluding the considerable dilatation usually associated with duodenal atresia.

An annular pancreas usually causes an *incomplete* obstruction of the second portion of the duodenum, thus permitting small, but recognizable, amounts of gas to pass into the gut distal to the duodenum. An annular pancreas will rarely cause a complete duodenal obstruction which will be associated with a roentgenological picture identical to that seen in this case. However, since the majority of the cases of annular pancreas seen in infants are only partially obstructing, one would not favor this diagnosis when confronted with the roentgen signs of complete obstruction as illustrated here (no gas distal to the markedly dilated stomach and duodenum). However, the tiny gas collections seen distal to a partly obstructed annular pancreas may be easily missed. Therefore, they should be carefully sought, since their presence excludes the diagnosis of duodenal atresia.

In the illustrations shown here the presence of the lumbar hemivertebra and the anomalies involving the posterior portions of the right fourth, fifth, and sixth ribs are not particularly helpful in differential diagnosis because such anomalies may be associated with *either* duodenal atresia or annular pancreas. Similarly, intestinal malrotation, Down's syndrome (mongolism), imperforate anus, and various urinary tract anomalies are seen in association with *both* duodenal atresia and annular pancreas, and are thus of little help in differentiating between these two conditions.

Normal rotation of the gut (Figures 17A, B, and C) usually precludes the development of midgut volvulus because of the broad mesenteric attachment of the small intestine (*dotted lines* in Figure 17C). Conversely, incomplete rotation results in a *narrow* mesenteric attachment (*dotted lines* in Figure 17D) of the small intestine which can, therefore, easily rotate around the axis of the superior mesenteric artery to cause midgut volvulus (Figure 17E). It is important to remember that incomplete rotation of the gut (Figure 17D) is an *associated* finding in approximately 20 per cent of all cases of congenital duodenal obstruction (duodenal atresia, duodenal diaphragm, duodenal stenosis, and annular pancreas). Therefore, since midgut volvulus is a dangerous complication of incomplete rotation of the intestine, and since incomplete rotation is a common associated finding in patients with congenital obstruction of the duodenum, it should always be considered as a *potential*, although not usually obvious, complicating factor when one sees roentgenologic evidence of duodenal obstruction in the newborn infant. Whenever a congenital obstruction of the duodenum is diagnosed, as on these illustrations, it is probably wise to do a barium enema to determine the position of the cecum. An abnormally located cecum (Figures 17D, E, F, and G) is a *most important* diagnostic roentgenologic finding because it indicates incomplete rotation which predisposes to the development of midgut volvulus (Figure 17E). The abnormally located cecum and ascending colon are usually in the mid abdomen or in the left side of the abdomen, the remainder of the colon usually being in normal position.

A small number of newborn infants with an abnormally placed cecum (malrotation) may also have dense congenital peritoneal bands ("Ladd's bands") which extend from the cecum or hepatic flexure over the anterior surface of the second or third portions of the duodenum (Figures 17F and G) to the right gutter and inferior surface of the liver. These dense bands can produce partial or complete obstruction of the second portion of the duodenum, in the latter event causing roentgenographic findings virtually identical to those of duodenal atresia. Some of these infants who have duodenal obstructions due to these bands also have associated midgut volvulus due to the associated malrotation. Since most cases of midgut volvulus (with or without such bands) are associated with malrotation and *partial obstruction*, gas and opaque contrast material can pass beyond the duodenum into the small intestine, thus precluding the presence of duodenal atresia.

If barium sulfate studies of the upper gastrointestinal tract are carried out after a barium enema has shown the abnormally positioned cecum, the nature of the duodenal obstruction (if present) can often be clearly defined. If barium passes such a partial obstruction, a "spiral" course of the midgut loops (Figure 17E) located in the right side of the abdomen will be highly suggestive of *midgut volvulus*. These findings in an infant whose duodenojejunal junction is located inferiorly and to the right of its expected position should be considered good evidence of midgut volvulus. Thus, before making a diagnosis of midgut volvulus in the newborn infant, it is understandable why many radiologists prefer to perform both barium enema and upper gastrointestinal studies. Conversely, since midgut volvulus may also occur as an unrecognized associated potentially fatal condition in infants who have the typical radiological manifestations of duodenal atresia (complete obstruction) as shown in this case, it should,

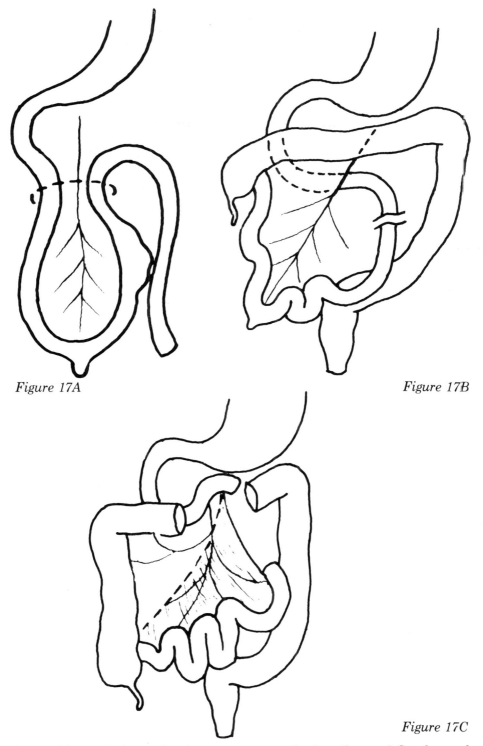

Figure 17A

Figure 17B

Figure 17C

Note: Many of these sketches are patterned after those of Snyder and Chaffin (see reference 5, "Midgut Volvulus", p. 102).

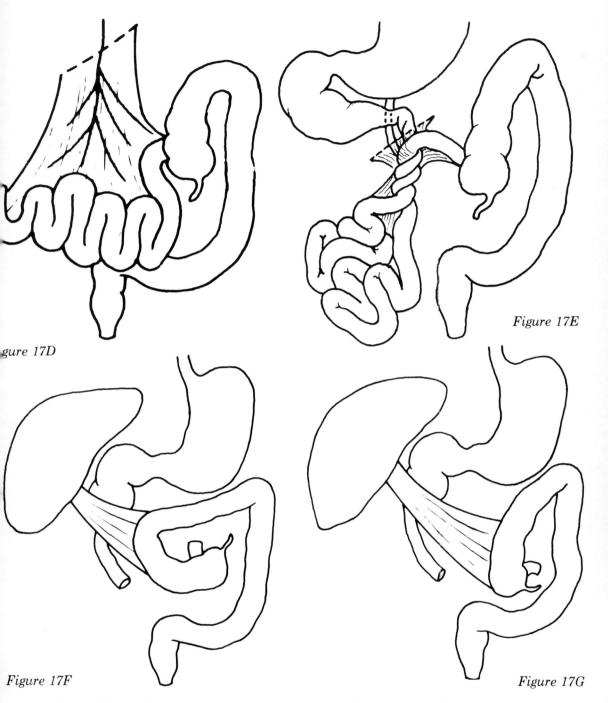

Figure 17E

Figure 17F

Figure 17G

Note: Many of these sketches are patterned after those of Snyder and Chaffin (see reference 5, "Midgut Volvulus", p. 102).

nevertheless, be suspected and a barium enema should be performed if the clinical condition of the infant indicates. It should also be remembered that esophageal atresia, with or without tracheoesophageal fistula, may occur in association with congenital duodenal obstructions. Therefore, roentgenograms of the abdomen should be carefully evaluated in infants who have tracheoesophageal fistulae in association with esophageal atresia. Conversely, the esophagus should probably be evaluated in all patients who have congenital duodenal obstruction.

Duodenal and gastric duplications of any type, either communicating or noncommunicating, are extremely rare causes of duodenal obstruction and do not show characteristic roentgen findings. On a statistical basis alone, a duplication would certainly not be the most likely diagnosis in the present case. Furthermore, most duodenal and gastric duplications are cyst-like structures filled with serous fluid, mucus, or even bile if the common bile duct empties into the cyst. Since they are usually located within the muscular layer of the duodenum (others may be submucous, subserous, or intramesenteric in location), they may encroach upon the lumen if they become large enough and will sometimes simulate a nonspecific intramural or extramural mass located on the inner aspect of the duodenum or lesser curvature or posterior wall of the stomach. Duplications rarely produce complete obstructions, and they are so infrequent compared to other causes of duodenal obstruction that such a diagnosis would be quite unlikely in the case shown here.

QUESTION 37

The correct answer to question 37 is (A). Duodenal atresia is more frequently associated with mongolism than any of the other possibilities listed in question 37.

QUESTION 38

The correct answer to question 38 is (D). All other listed answers are incorrect statements about congenital duodenal bands ("Ladd's bands"). These bands usually obstruct the *second* portion of the duodenum rather than the *first* part. They *are* usually associated with malrotation (Figures 17F and G) and because of this they *are* often present in patients who also have midgut volvulus. Such congenital bands do *not* cause meconium ileus which ensues as a result of obstruction by inspissated meconium located more distally in the small intestine.

QUESTION 39

Midgut volvulus is a condition which can occur *intermittently* throughout life and it is often spontaneously reversible and surprisingly benign in its clinical manifestations. It often corrects itself (untwists) without surgical intervention. Therefore, **the correct answer to question 39 is (B)** because it is the *only* incorrect statement among those listed as possible responses. All other possible answers listed are *true* statements about midgut volvulus.

QUESTION 40

The correct answer to question 40 is (A) because annular pancreas is more frequently discovered in *adults* than in children. Most cases do not produce obstruction during infancy, childhood, or adulthood. Thus, in most patients with this condition there are minimal symptoms. It is the rare case which produces such a high grade of obstruction in newborn infants. All other answers in question 40 are *true* statements about annular pancreas.

In summary, the characteristic "double bubble" appearance *without evidence* of any intraluminal gas distal to the bulb, is due to duodenal atresia in the vast majority of instances for the reasons mentioned earlier. Even small amounts of gas distal to a duodenal obstruction usually indicate the presence of an annular pancreas or midgut volvulus and preclude the presence of duodenal atresia which is associated with *complete* obstruction. In newborn infants with the roentgen findings of a duodenal obstruction, the presence of intestinal malrotation and midgut volvulus should always be considered possible, particularly if surgical interference is *not immediately contemplated*. Conversely, if an operation is done promptly to relieve the duodenal obstruction, the associated possibility of infarction of the entire small intestine due to midgut volvulus can then be evaluated and treated.

SUGGESTED READINGS

DUODENAL ATRESIA

1. Caffey J: *Pediatric X-Ray Diagnosis, Vol 2*, 6th ed, pp 1486, 1495–1499. Year Book Medical Publishers, Chicago, 1972
2. Faegenburg D, Bosniak M: Duodenal anomalies in the adult. Am J Roentgenol *88*:642–657, 1962
3. Fonkalsrud EW, DeLorimier AA, Hays DM: Congenital atresia and stenosis of the duodenum. A review compiled from the members of the surgical section of the American Academy of Pediatrics. Pediatrics *43*:79–83, 1969

ANNULAR PANCREAS

1. Free EA, Gerald B: Duodenal obstruction in the newborn due to annular pancreas. Am J Roentgenol *103*:321–329, 1968
2. Hope JW, Gibbons JF: Duodenal obstruction due to annular pancreas with a

differential diagnosis of other congenital lesions producing duodenal obstruction. Radiology 63:473–490, 1954.

3. Lundquist G: Annular pancreas. Pathogenesis, clinical features, and treatment with report on two operation cases. Acta Chir Scandinav 117:451–464, 1959

MIDGUT VOLVULUS

1. Berdon WE, Baker DH, Bull S, Santulli TV: Midgut malrotation and volvulus. Which films are most helpful? Radiology 96:375–383, 1970
2. Caffey J: *Pediatric X-Ray Diagnosis, Vol 1*, 6th ed, pp 645–647. Yeak Book Medical Publishers, Chicago, 1972
3. Houston CS, Wittenborg MH: Roentgen evaluation of anomalies of rotation and fixation of the bowel in children. Radiology 84:1–18, 1965
4. Singleton EG: Radiologic evaluation of intestinal obstruction in the newborn. Radiol Clin North Am 1:571–581, 1963
5. Snyder WH, Chaffin L: Malrotation of the intestine. In CB Benson, WT Mustard, MM Ravitch, WH Snyder, KJ Welch: *Pediatric Surgery, Vol. 2*, pp. 683–691. Year Book Medical Publishers, Chicago, 1969

DUODENAL BAND

1. Berdon WE, Baker DH, Bull S, Santulli TV: Midgut malrotation and volvulus. Which films are most helpful? Radiology 96:375–383, 1970
2. Faegenburg D, Bosniak M: Duodenal anomalies in the adult. Am J Roentgenol 88:642–657, 1962
3. Ladd WE: Congenital obstruction of the duodenum. New England J Med 206: 277–283, 1932

CORRECT ANSWERS

Question 36-(B)
Question 37-(A)
Question 38-(D)
Question 39-(B)
Question 40-(A)

NOTES

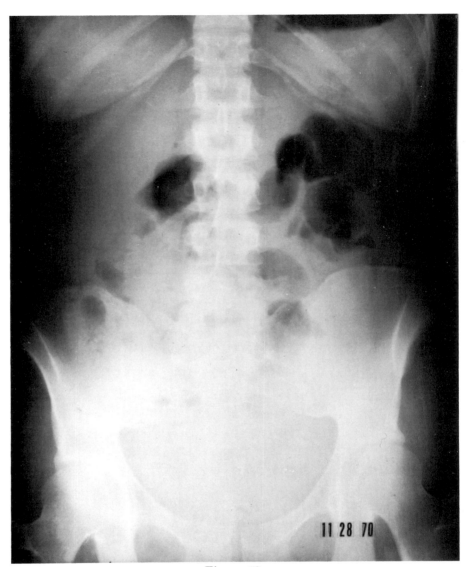

Figure 18

Figures 18, 19, and 20. This 20-year-old woman complains of 3 days of
progressively increasing cramping abdominal pain, 4 weeks after an uncomplicated delivery of a normal infant. Roentgenograms were taken with
the patient in the supine position (Figure 18) on the night of admission to
the hospital, and in the supine (Figure 19) and upright (Figure 20) positions 3 days later.

Questions 41 through 46

41. Which one of the following is the *MOST* likely diagnosis?

    (A) Twisted ovarian cyst
    (B) Pseudocyst of the pancreas
    (C) Small bowel obstruction
    (D) Tubo-ovarian abscess
    (E) Massive ascites

For each of the numbered clinical disorders listed below (Questions 42—46), select the *one* lettered roentgenographic sign (A,B,C,D,E) that is *MOST* closely associated with it. Each lettered roentgenographic sign may be selected once, more than once, or not at all.

    (A) "Pseudotumor"
    (B) "Football"
    (C) "Ground glass"
    (D) "Coffee bean"
    (E) "Dog ear"

42. Sigmoid volvulus

43. Strangulating small bowel obstruction

44. Pneumoperitoneum

45. Ascites

46. Pelvic fluid

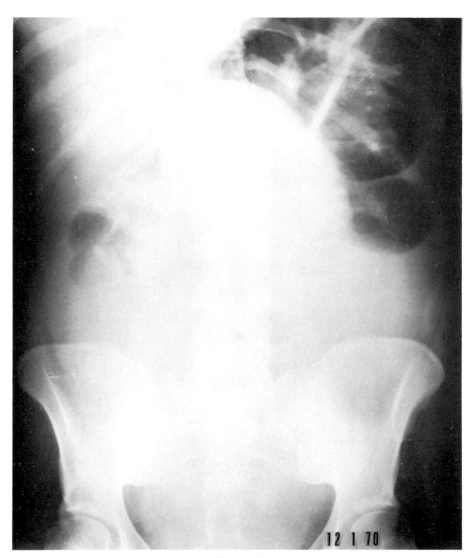

Figure 19

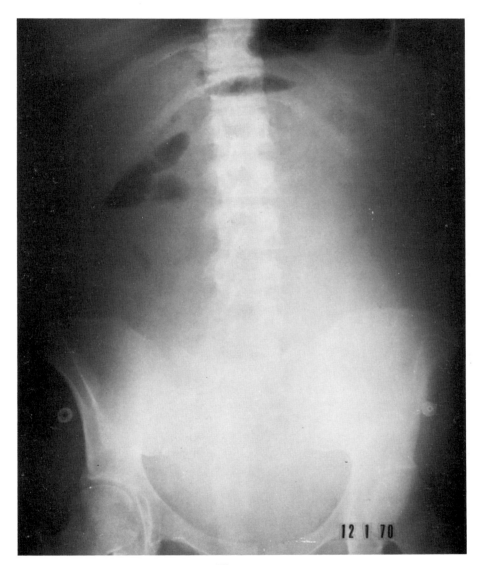

Figure 20

Discussion

This is a more obvious than usual example of the "pseudotumor" sign associated with a small bowel obstruction. **The correct diagnosis in this case is therefore (C).** In *simple* mechanical small bowel obstruction swallowed air leads to gaseous distention of the small bowel loops characteristically seen on supine and upright roentgenograms. Distention of the intestine, in turn, causes an out-pouring of fluid into the lumen. If the fluid and gas are evenly distributed in the bowel proximal to the obstruction, characteristic multiple fluid levels or a "stepladder" appearance are seen on the upright view. If, however, a segment of the intestinal tract is occluded at *both* ends and cannot receive gas through the proximal obstructed point, then the continued out-pouring of fluid into what is a relatively "closed-loop" will result in marked distention of this loop into an almost cystic structure. Such a loop may frequently contain small amounts of gas as is evident at the top of the large roundish mass seen on erect films (Figure 20B, below *broken line*). Such a "closed-loop" may contain no gas if the latter happens to have been absorbed prior to the development of massive distention or if none has entered this segment of bowel after the development of obstruction. The presence of such a large, homogeneous, usually reasonably well-defined, water-density mass on films made during the study of the "acute abdomen" is an important sign of small bowel obstruction, serving as a warning of strangulation (constriction of vascular supply of an intestinal loop or loops usually due to twisting, but sometimes due to severe stretching or other compression of the mesenteric attachment of the bowel loop). This deprivation of blood supply leads to necrosis and thus to perforation and peritonitis.

The "pseudotumor" outline may be seen on the films of patients with acute small bowel obstruction at the time of admission. As in this case, the lesion sometimes may become more apparent over a period of time due to the continued passage of fluid into the lumen of the involved loop.

As far as the differential diagnosis is concerned, it is doubtful that a twisted ovarian cyst could have increased to this size during 60 hours without rupturing. Otherwise, a twisted ovarian cyst would be an important differential diagnostic consideration when acute abdominal symptoms and roentgen findings of this type are present.

Pseudocysts of the pancreas are generally found higher in the abdomen and ordinarily would cause local displacement of the gas-containing upper abdominal hollow viscera (stomach, transverse colon, and upper small bowel). Also, while pancreatic pseudocysts can become remarkably large, the lesion in this case is larger than any pseudocysts the authors have seen. Due to the surrounding inflammatory response, pancreatic pseudocysts are usually not as well defined (Figure 20A, *arrows*) as is the mass in this case. While pancreatic pseudocysts, especially those developing after trauma to the upper abdomen, can develop rapidly, development to this size in a matter of 3 days would be most unlikely.

The diagnosis of tubo-ovarian abscess is unlikely because a tubo-ovarian abscess will not reach this size without rupture and because abscesses are rarely as sharply demarcated from surrounding tissues. Thus, the sharp margin along the upper portion of the mass projected to the left of the upper lumbar spine (Figure 20A, *arrows*) is against the diagnosis of abscess.

The last differential diagnosis, massive ascites, is made unlikely by the distribution of the fluid. One ordinarily does not find sharp outlines (as in the left upper quadrant in this case) with ascites. Also, the gas-containing intestinal loops in patient with ascites are found in the *middle* of the abdomen in contrast to the paucity of centrally located gas shadows in this case. The highest point in the abdomen in the supine patient is near the midline and the floating, gas-containing loops often congregate there in the presence of ascites. The fluid-containing mass in this case also has impressed itself upon the bowel loops in the upper abdomen in a manner unlikely to be caused by free intraperitoneal fluid. It is also notable that the fluid-containing loops of bowel seen here do not sag downward in the upright position as much as would be expected of free ascitic fluid. In fact, the failure of an appreciable change in position of such a "tumor" when the patient changes from the recumbent to an upright position is in itself *suggestive* of a strangulating obstruction, because it indicates *fixation* of a large mass which would otherwise move noticeably toward the most dependent part of the peritoneal cavity. In this case, note that the top of the mass (*broken lines* in Figures 20A and B) remains in virtually the *same* relationship to the centrum of T-11 on both the supine and erect roentgenograms. Many strangulated obstructions of the "closed-loop" type, whether due to internal herniation through holes in a broad ligament, the mesentery, or omentum, or due to adhesive bands, or volvulus, will remain relatively *fixed* in location, even though roentgenograms have been made in different positions.

It is fairly characteristic that a discrete "mass" of fluid-filled loops of small intestine cannot be palpated, even though a solid tumor appears to be present on the roentgenograms. Thus, the term "pseudotumor" seems appropriate from both the clinical and roentgen standpoints.

Although it is routine to correct any fluid and electrolyte deficiencies as

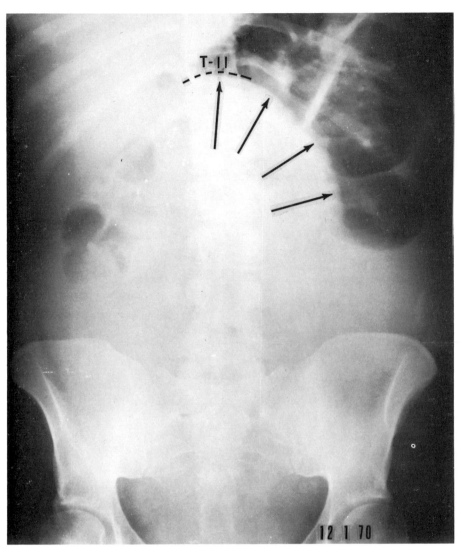

Figure 20A

quickly as possible and to remedy intestinal obstruction promptly, the major importance of recognizing the "pseudotumor" sign is that it enables the radiologist to alert the referring physician to the likelihood that *strangulation* is developing. This is a far more urgent indication for operation than is the presence of simple bowel obstruction.

Patients with strangulating obstruction often have signs of peritoneal irritation. However, the absence of such signs is of only limited value in deciding on the timing of operative intervention. This patient was operated

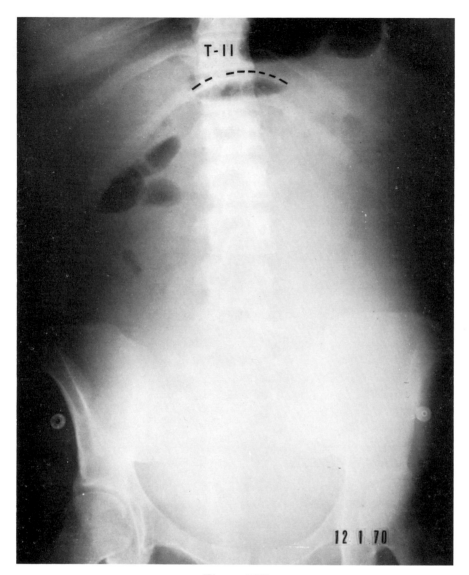

Figure 20B

upon immediately after the roentgenograms showed the "pseudotumor". Even at that time a 40 cm. long segment of strangulated dead bowel had to be resected, having been incarcerated as a result of its passage through an opening created under a large adhesion which extended from the cecum to the root of the mesentery of the small intestine.

In addition to the above listed findings, Rack and Glazer suggest that a hazy or "ground glass" appearance of an area with a sometimes lobulated outline may be suggestive of strangulation; i.e., the increased permeability of these loops results in the leaking of fluid both to the inside and the *outside* of the lumen, thus creating the roentgen picture of a poorly defined hazy water-density mass.

It is characteristic for a strangulating type of obstruction to be associated with a steadily rising white blood count with a predominance of polymorphonuclear leukocytes. The white blood count will often rise to 20,000 to 30,000 per mm.[3] Shock and severe abdominal pain are common. Nausea, vomiting, and crampng abdominal pain are characteristic of *simple nonstrangulating* types of small bowel obstruction and of obstruction of other smooth muscle organs (bile ducts, ureters). However, the pain with strangulation is more severe and continuous than that associated with nonstrangulating obstruction. High fever, although sometimes seen in patients with strangulating obstruction, occurs in other conditions as well and is, therefore, not diagnostic by itself.

The following are the associations of named signs with clinical disorders as used in common radiological practice:

QUESTION 42

The correct answer to question 42 is (D). The "coffee bean" sign is produced by an intestinal loop sharply reflected on itself and containing gas. It is most characteristically seen in volvulus of the sigmoid colon, but a similar appearance may at times be seen in twisted small bowel loops.

QUESTION 43

The correct answer to question 43 is (A). "Pseudotumor", as has just been discussed, is an indication of strangulating intestinal obstruction. (Incidentally, in chest roentgen diagnosis this term refers to a localized intrafissural fluid collection.)

QUESTION 44

The correct answer to question 44 is (B). The "football" sign (see discussion on p. 156) is a descriptive term referring to the configuration of a large pneumoperitoneum as seen on supine films of the abdomen. In the presence of perforated stomach or bowel a large amount of free peritoneal air will often outline the *entire* peritoneal cavity, the overall contour of which often resembles the outline of a football. The falciform ligament, (see Figures 30A and B, *small black horizontal arrows*, pp. 158–159) made visible by intraperitoneal air surrounding it, suggests one of the seams on a football.

QUESTION 45

The correct answer to question 45 is (C). The "ground glass" sign, seen in massive ascites, results from loss of visibility of organ outlines in the abdominal cavity owing to a dimunition of roentgenographic contrast which, in turn, is due to the increased amount of water-density material (ascitic fluid) which must be penetrated by the roentgen ray beam, and the associated invisibility of the fat planes due to their infiltration with water-density edema fluid.

QUESTION 46

The correct answer to question 46 is (E). "Dog ears", a term particularly emphasized by McCort, indicates the accumulation of fluid in the lesser pelvis, especially in the recesses around and behind the bladder, and between the bladder and the lower small bowel loops.

SUGGESTED READINGS

ACUTE ABDOMEN, GENERAL

Bryk D, Rosenkranz W: Functional evaluation of the acute abdomen by radiological means. CRC Crit Rev Radiol Sci 2:1–45, 1971

STRANGULATING OBSTRUCTION

1. Mellins HZ, Rigler LG: The roentgen findings in strangulating obstructions of the small intestine. Am J Roentgenol 71:404–415, 1954
2. Rack RJ, Glazer N: A suggestive x-ray sign of strangulation in intestinal obstruction. Arch Surg 69:233–214, 1954
3. Rigler LG, Pogue WL: Roentgen signs of intestinal necrosis. Am J Roentgenol 94:402–409, 1965
4. Shauffer IA, Ferris EJ: The mass sign in primary volvulus of the small intestine in adults. Radiology 94:374–378, 1965
5. Tomchik FS, Wittenberg J, Ottinger LW: The roentgenographic spectrum of bowel infarction. Radiology 96:249–260, 1970
6. Williams JL: Fluid-filled loops in intestinal obstruction. Am J Roentgenol 88:677–687, 1962

PNEUMOPERITONEUM

Miller RE: Perforated viscus in infants: a new roentgen sign. Radiology 74:65–67, 1960

ASCITES

Keeffe EJ, Gagliardi RA, Pfister RC: The roentgenographic evaluation of ascites. Am J Roentgenol 101:388–396, 1967

PELVIC FLUID

McCort JJ: Radiologic examination in blunt abdominal trauma. Radiol Clin North Am 2:121–143, 1964

CORRECT ANSWERS

Question 41-(C)
Question 42-(D)
Question 43-(A)
Question 44-(B)
Question 45-(C)
Question 46-(E)

NOTES

NOTES

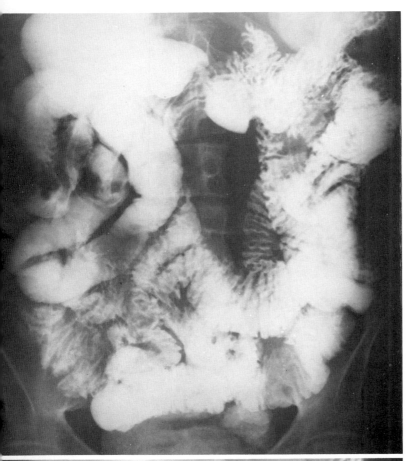

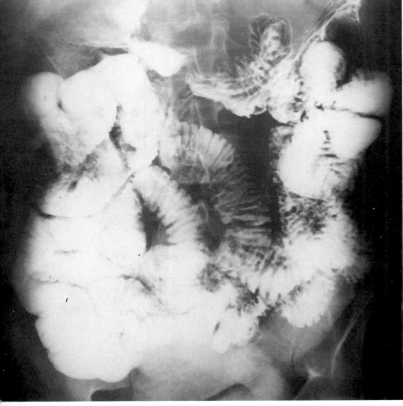

Figures 21 (top), 22 (bottom), 23 and 24. This 41-year-old man has a 1-year history of vague abdominal discomfort and loss of appetite. Figures 21 and 22 are roentgenograms taken during a small bowel study, and Figures 23 and 24 are close-up views.

Questions 47 through 54

47. Which one of the following is the *MOST* likely diagnosis?

    (A) Sprue
    (B) Regional enteritis
    (C) Scleroderma
    (D) Whipple's disease
    (E) Zollinger-Ellison syndrome

For each of the numbered disease entities listed below (Questions 48–52), select the *one* lettered feature (A,B,C,D,E) that is *MOST* closely associated with it. Each lettered feature may be selected once, more than once, or not at all.

    (A) "Creeping fat"
    (B) "Pseudo-obstruction"
    (C) Arthralgia
    (D) Peptic ulceration of the jejunum
    (E) "Moulage"

48. Sprue

49. Regional enteritis

50. Scleroderma

51. Whipple's disease

52. Zollinger-Ellison syndrome

53. Which one of the following is *LEAST* likely to occur in sprue?

    (A) Intussusception
    (B) Mucosal atrophy
    (C) Segmentation
    (D) Ulceration
    (E) Widening of mucosal folds

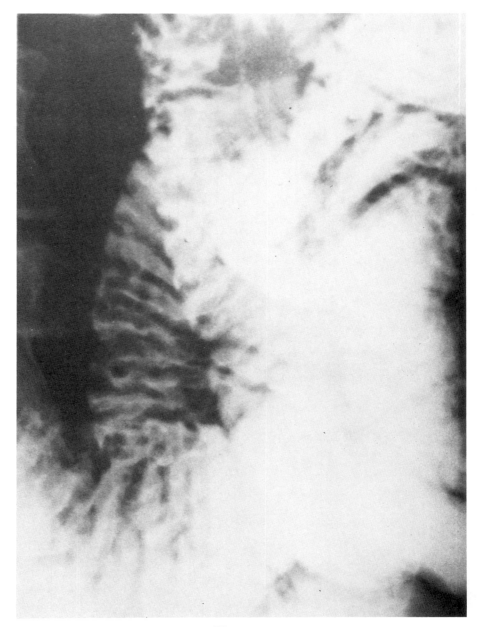

Figure 23

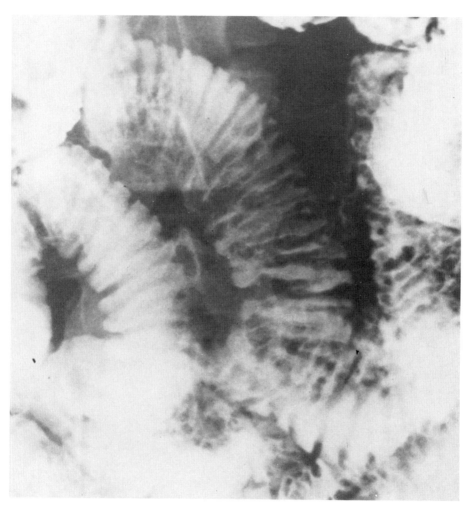

Figure 24

54. Which one of the following prognostic statements concerning Whipple's disease is *MOST* likely?

(A) It is always progressive in spite of therapy
(B) A gluten-free diet is the best treatment
(C) Antibiotics can produce cure
(D) Resection of the diseased jejunum is advisable
(E) None of the above

Discussion

QUESTION 47

The correct answer to question 47 is (D). As in most cases of Whipple's disease, the roentgenograms illustrated here show a mild but fairly widespread dilatation of the small bowel without obstruction. Furthermore, there is moderate thickening of the mucosal folds in the jejunum which have *small protuberances* or nodules on them (Figures 24A and B, *arrows*). The dilatation and slight prominence of jejunal folds in themselves are not typical of Whipple's disease, but the small *nodules* on the folds are highly suggestive, especially when the changes are limited to the jejunum. On these films and on subsequent followup films, the ileum appears normal except for a mild dilatation.

Sprue generally is associated with a less well defined contour of the mucosal folds and, if anything, in sprue there are changes of atrophy rather than fold enlargement. Furthermore, the small nodular excrescences seen here are not seen in sprue. Also, in sprue there is ordinarily much more intraluminal fluid and segmentation of the barium column.

Regional enteritis is one of the entities which is most difficult to differentiate from Whipple's disease because early regional enteritis with some degree of edema may appear very similar to the changes illustrated here. However, one would not expect to see the clearly defined nodularity seen in this case, although in regional enteritis, the thickened folds may be slightly irregular in contour. Furthermore, while regional enteritis can present in any portion of the intestinal tract, it usually is more pronounced or first appears in the distal portion of the small bowel in contrast to Whipple's disease which is most frequently limited to the jejunum.

Scleroderma, when affecting the small bowel, shows a rather marked dilatation of the upper small bowel with marked delay of transit of the contrast material ("pseudo-obstruction"). The folds in the dilated small intestine in scleroderma are usually sharply defined, straight, and of normal thickness, in contrast to the thickening, irregularity, and nodularity seen in Whipple's disease. Occasionally, in scleroderma, the esophagus will contain barium for a long time after the performance of the study due to the interference with the propulsive mechanism of this organ. This finding may help give a clue to the correct diagnosis in scleroderma.

The Zollinger-Ellison syndrome is not a likely diagnosis in this case due to the fact that we observe none of the characteristic findings of that disease; i.e., enlargement of the gastric folds, hypersecretions, peptic ulcers in the region of the ligament of Treitz (Figure 10B, *top white arrow*, p. 60), edema of the jejunal mucosal folds (Figure 10C, *arrows*, p. 61), or dilution of the barium in the small bowel ("*X*" in Figures 10G and H, p. 64).

QUESTION 48

The correct answer to question 48 is (E) since sprue is associated with the "moulage" sign. The term implies moulding or casting and implies an unusually good conformation of the barium to the contour of the intestinal loop. Possibly, this appearance could be due to the atrophy of mucosal folds which occurs in sprue with resultant unindented margins of the barium filled loops due to the absence of the normal indentations of the folds. We have found that segmentation of the barium column and the large accumulation of fluid in the moderately dilated small intestine are more characteristic of sprue and more readily explained than is the "moulage" sign.

QUESTION 49

The correct answer to question 49 is (A) since regional enteritis is the only listed condition associated with "creeping fat". This descriptive term refers to the gross appearance of the bowel when inspected at operation or during a study of the specimen. Due to the chronic inflammatory process and probable obstruction of the small bowel lymphatic drainage, there is a tendency for fat to accumulate in the lymphatics which drain from the small intestine into the mesentery. This fat often accumulates on the mesenteric side of the small intestine and appears to "creep" onto the contiguous mesentery. Hence the diagnostic term "creeping fat". This gross pathological finding is probably one of the earliest changes of regional enteritis and occurs at about the same time that the radiologist can recognize the earliest roentgen changes; i.e., enlarged edematous folds.

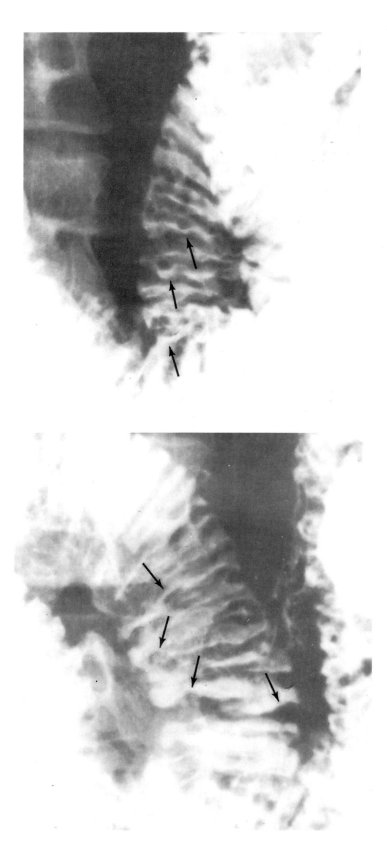

Figures 24A (top) and B (bottom)

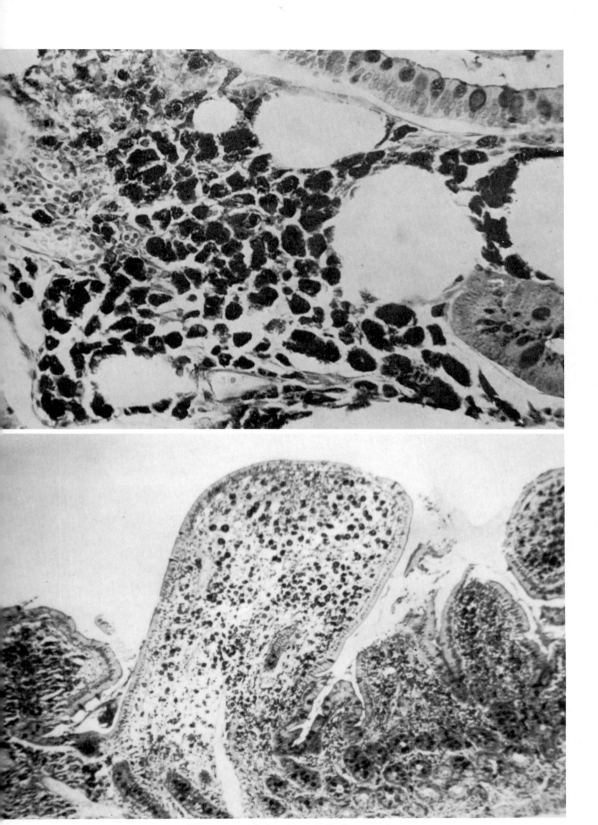

Figures 24C (top) and D (bottom)

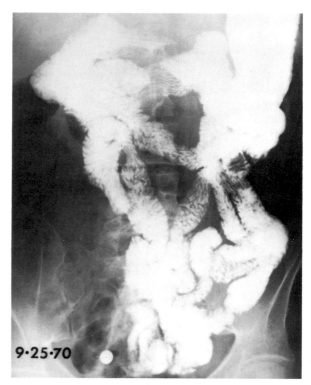

9·25·70

Figure 24E

QUESTION 50

The correct answer to question 50 is (B) since scleroderma is associated with one type of "pseudo-obstruction". The term "pseudo-obstruction" has been applied to a number of different conditions of the intestine in which dilatation on either the plain films or barium studies suggests obstruction, even though the lumen is not truly obstructed. In scleroderma the association of the markedly dilated somewhat atonic upper small bowel with a severe delay in the passage of barium is quite suggestive of obstruction, and the term "pseudo-obstruction" is indeed an appropriate one.

QUESTION 51

The correct answer to question 51 is (C) since Whipple's disease is characteristically associated with arthralgia as part of the systemic changes of this disease. None of the other possible answers is relevant to Whipple's disease.

QUESTION 52

The correct answer to question 52 is (D) since peptic ulceration of the jejunum is virtually diagnostic of the Zollinger-Ellison syndrome. As a matter of fact, the first cases described by Zollinger and Ellison in 1955 both showed the development of jejunal ulcers as part of what at first appeared to be unusually stubborn cases of recurrent ulcer disease after conventional operations for peptic ulcer disease.

QUESTION 53

The correct answer to question 53 is (D) since all of the other statements are descriptions of findings which *do* occur in sprue. Sprue, however, is not an ulcerating disease and the development of obvious ulcers would be unlikely.

QUESTION 54

The correct answer to question 54 is (C). Antibiotics can produce cure in most cases of Whipple's disease. Until the development of antibiotic treatment, Whipple's disease was indeed quite resistant to treatment. However, it is now known that antibiotics can produce complete reversal of the symptoms and findings as was true in the case presented here (see Figure 24E for normal appearance of this patient's small intestine 9 months after original films). It is not quite clear whether this is in fact a permanent cure or whether the disease will recur later. A gluten free diet is appropriate treatment for sprue, but not for Whipple's disease, although malabsorption may be a secondary problem in Whipple's disease. Operative treatment is not indicated in view of the success of antibiotic therapy and the notable lack of success of surgical treatment.

DISCUSSION

Whipple's disease is an uncommon disease affecting primarily the upper small bowel. A most striking feature is the accumulation of macrophages in the intestinal submucosa, as well as in other tissues. These macrophages contain material which stains positively with the periodic acid-Schiff (PAS) stain. Electron microscopic studies suggest that this material is bacterial in origin. Bacterial structures are also found between the cells. Figure 24C shows the PAS-positive granular material in large macrophages (the *dark structures* in this illustration). The large round clear spaces are dilated lymphatics. Figure 24D is a lower magnification overview of a markedly enlarged villus which almost appears to be "distended" with macrophages containing the dense PAS-positive material (*dark structures* in Figure 24D). Note the single layer of columnar epithelium on the surface of this bulbous swollen microvillus. The width of this microvillus is about four times that of a normal microvillus. If the hundreds of microvilli projecting from the surface of each of the thousands of villi on each mucosal fold are enlarged to this degree, it can be understood why each mucosal fold becomes enlarged in Whipple's disease. The distention of the lymphatics (Figure 24C, *clear spaces*) also contributes to the balloon-like distention of some of the villi which may account for some of the small nodules seen on the mucosal folds in Whipple's disease (Figures 24A and B, *arrows*). Although Whipple's disease in many respects resembles a reticuloendotheliosis, the present evidence favors a bacterial origin. A less likely hypothesis is that the PAS-positive bacterial material is the *result*, rather than the *cause*, of this disease. Antibiotics must be given for long periods of time because regression of the changes is rather slow. In this case, the small bowel had returned to a normal radiographic appearance after 9 months of antibiotic therapy (compare Figures 21 and 22 with Figure 24E).

An interesting feature of the disease is the previously mentioned dilatation of the lymphatics in the bowel wall and on its surface. The dilated lymphatics which are obvious microscopically (*round clear areas* in Figure 24B), contain fatty material. The mesenteric lymph nodes are also enlarged and soft and it is possible that the low grade inflammatory changes in these nodes might cause lymph stasis due to partial obstruction to the flow of lymph from the small bowel through the nodes. Lymph nodes elsewhere in the body may also be enlarged. Eventually considerable fibrotic changes may develop in the involved areas.

While the typical initial roentgen manifestations of Whipple's disease consist simply of some thickening of the mucosal folds with nodularity as shown on these illustrations (Figures 24A and B, *arrows*), there may be minimal or no dilatation. These changes are restricted primarily to the jejunum. There may occasionally be roentgen changes suggesting malabsorption (excessive fluid), in addition to the dilatation and large folds as seen here. In such cases it would be difficult if not impossible to distinguish Whipple's disease from sprue. One of the major ways in which Whipple's disease differs from sprue is that there is no nodularity of the mucosal folds in sprue and there is usually rather considerable dilatation in sprue. Another lesion which is difficult to differentiate radiographically from Whipple's disease is lymphangiectasia. However, lymphangiectasia usually involves the entire bowel rather than just the jejunum.

In a few cases of Whipple's disease roentgen findings have been described in the colon. It may sometimes even be possible to make the diagnosis by rectal biopsy.

A host of other diseases (*not* listed as possible answers here) can cause small bowel changes which may be virtually impossible to differentiate from Whipple's disease; i.e., lymphoid hyperplasia of various types, macroglobulinemia, and hypogammaglobulinemia. Furthermore, other lesions such as angioneurotic or other types of edema, and lymphoma should be considered in the diagnostic process. While a presumptive roentgen diagnosis can often be made, a definite diagnosis frequently requires small bowel biopsy and careful consideration of clinical and laboratory data because of the close similarity of many of these lesions.

SUGGESTED READINGS

SPRUE

Marshak RH, Lindner AE: *Radiology of the Small Intestine*, pp 11–29. WB Saunders Co, Philadelphia, 1970

REGIONAL ENTERITIS

Marshak RH, Lindner, RE: *Radiology of the Small Intestine*, pp 158–222 WB Saunders Co, Philadelphia, 1970

SCLERODERMA—"PSEUDO-OBSTRUCTION"

1. Hale CH, Schatzki R: The roentgenological appearance of the gastrointestinal tract in scleroderma. Am J Roentgenol *51:*407–420, 1944
2. Peachy RD, Creamer B, Pierce JW: Sclerodermatous involvement of the stomach and small and large bowel. Gut *10:*285–292, 1969
3. Treachy WL, Bounting WL, Gambill EE, Code CF: Scleroderma presenting as obstruction of the small bowel. Proc Staff Meetings Mayo Clinic *37:*607–616, 1962

WHIPPLE'S DISEASE (also see bibliography on p. 68)

1. Clemett AR, Marshak RH: Whipple's disease. Roentgen features and differential diagnosis. Radiol Clin North Am *7:*105–111, 1969
2. Rice RP, Roufail W, Reeves RJ: The roentgen diagnosis of Whipple's disease (intestinal lipodystrophy) with emphasis on improvement following antibiotic therapy. Radiology *88:*295–301, 1967
3. Whipple GH: A hitherto undescribed disease characterized anatomically by deposits of fat and fatty acids in the intestinal and mesenteric lymphatic tissues. Bull Johns Hopkins Hosp *18:*382–391, 1907
4. Yardley JH, Hendrix TR: Combined electron and light microscopy in Whipple's disease. Bull Johns Hopkins Hosp *109:*80–98, 1961

DIFFERENTIAL DIAGNOSIS OF WHIPPLE'S DISEASE

1. Hodgson JR, Hoffman HN II, Huizenga KA: Roentgenologic features of lymphoid hyperplasia of the small intestine associated with dysgammaglobulinemia. Radiology *88:*883–888, 1967
2. Khilnani MT, Keller RJ, Cuttner J: Macroglobulinemia and steatorrhea: roentgen and pathologic findings in the intestinal tract. Radiol Clin North Am *7:*43–55, 1969
3. Person KD, Buchignani JS, Shimkin PM, Frank MM: Hereditary angioneurotic edema of the gastrointestinal tract. Am J Roentgenol *116:*256–261, 1972
4. Theros EG: RPC of the month from the A.F.I.P. Radiology *92:*1363–1368, 1969

5. Vermess M, Waldmann TA, Person KD: Radiographic manifestations of primary acquired hypogammaglobulinemia. Radiology *107:* 63–69, 1973

ZOLLINGER-ELLISON SYNDROME

See bibliography on page 67

CORRECT ANSWERS

Question 47-(D)
Question 48-(E)
Question 49-(A)
Question 50-(B)
Question 51-(C)
Question 52-(D)
Question 53-(D)
Question 54-(C)

NOTES

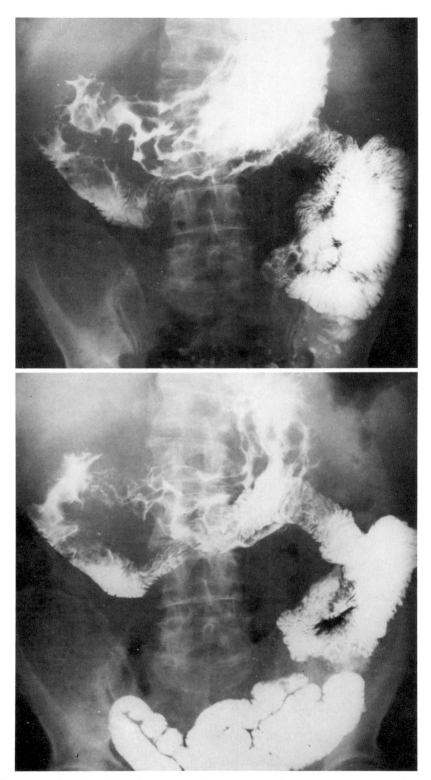

Figures 25 (top) and 26 (bottom). This 65-year-old man has a 1-year history of malaise, poor appetite, and abdominal fullness. You are shown two roentgenograms taken during an upper GI series.

Questions 55 through 58

55. Which one of the following is the *MOST* likely diagnosis?

    (A) Giant hypertrophic gastritis
    (B) Zollinger-Ellison syndrome
    (C) Superficial spreading carcinoma
    (D) Lymphosarcoma
    (E) Eosinophilic gastroenteritis

56. Which one of the following is *MOST* commonly associated with giant hypertrophic gastritis?

    (A) Multiple ulcers
    (B) Islet cell tumor of the pancreas
    (C) Excessive gastric secretion
    (D) Gastric bleeding
    (E) Involvement mainly of the lesser curvature

57. In the differential diagnosis between the Zollinger-Ellison syndrome and gastrointestinal lymphoma, which one of the following roentgenographic findings is *MOST* suggestive of the Zollinger-Ellison syndrome?

    (A) Multiple ulcerations
    (B) Gastric hypersecretion
    (C) Retrogastric mass
    (D) Enlargement of the gastric mucosal folds
    (E) Abnormal small bowel mucosal pattern

58. Which one of the following statements about eosinophilic gastroenteritis is *LEAST* likely?

    (A) Usually the entire stomach is involved
    (B) It is not premalignant
    (C) It is not related to granuloma with eosinophils
    (D) A history of allergy is usually present
    (E) A peripheral eosinophilia is frequently seen

Discussion

QUESTION 55

The correct answer to question 55 is (D). Diffuse infiltration of the gastric mucosal folds, resulting in their enlargement, is one of the manifestations of lymphoma of the stomach. The enlarged folds in this case apparently involve all or a large part of the stomach. Although enlarged, the folds are well defined, the stomach changes in size and contour (compare Figure 25 to Figure 26), excessive secretions are *not* evident, and there are similar mucosal pattern changes in the first and second portions of the duodenum (Figure 26A, *small arrows*). These films do not permit a clear-cut evaluation of the thickness of the gastric wall, although there is some suggestion (Figure 26A, *large arrows*) that the wall of the body of the stomach on the greater curvature side is thickened. The distance from the faintly seen thin layer of serosal fat (Figure 26A, *two lowest large arrows*) to the intragastric barium sometimes permits an estimation of the thickness of the wall of the stomach. Note that a few small streaks of barium extend from the lumen into the apparent thick gastric wall, much of the volume of which is comprised of the large folds which are crowded together in the somewhat contracted stomach (Figure 26A).

Of the differential diagnostic possibilities listed, giant hypertrophic gastritis is probably the most difficult to exclude. While in many cases of giant hypertrophic gastritis there is marked hypersecretion and loss of protein from the intestinal tract, hypertrophic gastritis can occur without such excessive secretions. The somewhat lumpy, localized involvement of the duodenum in this case would serve to rule out ordinary hypertrophic gastritis, since the duodenal folds are not enlarged in this condition.

The Zollinger-Ellison syndrome is also unlikely because of the absence of increased secretions and absence of identifiable ulceration. In fact, the gastric mucosa appears surprisingly "dry" because of the absence of significant amounts of fluid. Superficial spreading carcinoma is restricted to the stomach and also is usually a localized lesion in contrast to the diffuse gastric involvement seen here. Furthermore, extensive enlargement of folds is one of the less frequent manifestations of superficial spreading carcinoma of the stomach, the more common changes including ulceration, evidence of mass, and antral deformity. Eosinophilic gastroenteritis is an unusual condition associated with small bowel involvement, malabsorption, and protein loss. Its roentgen appearance, however, suggests gastric fold atrophy rather than enlargement as seen in this case. Furthermore, the involvement is

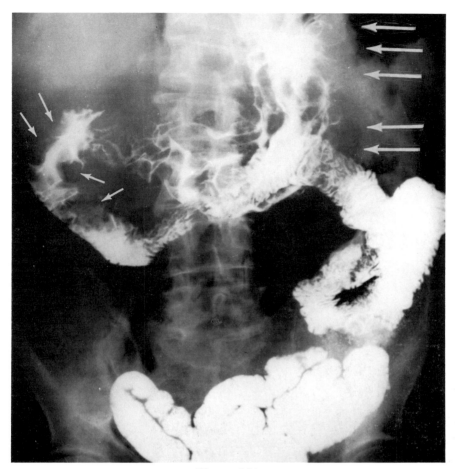

Figure 26A

typically limited to the *distal* portion of the stomach, presenting an irregular gastric outline with antral or pyloric narrowing. In eosinophilic gastro-enteritis, eosinophilic infiltration is found in the submucosa, muscularis, and serosa of the stomach and small bowel with relative sparing of the mucosa.

QUESTION 56

The correct answer to question 56 is (C). Of all the possible answers listed, the one most commonly associated with giant hypertrophic gastritis is excessive gastric secretions. Giant hypertrophy of the gastric mucosal folds (their enlargement is not closely related to histological inflammatory changes) can occur as an isolated lesion, although large folds may be associated with an islet cell tumor of the pancreas (the Zollinger-Ellison syndrome) or other assorted causes to be discussed later. In the Zollinger-Ellison syndrome there is usually ulceration, frequently in the form of ordinary peptic ulcer disease of duodenum but also in the jejunum or the stomach. Conversely, giant hypertrophic gastritis is not in itself an ulcerating disease. Gastric bleeding is not characteristic of giant hypertrophic gastritis in contrast to superficial erosive gastritis in which disease it is often massive. Enlargement of the gastric folds, especially if associated with hypersecretion, loss of protein from the intestinal tract, and hypoproteinemia is known as Menetrier's syndrome. The enlargement of the folds in this condition is usually most obvious along the greater curvature of the stomach, whereas it is *not* characteristic along the lesser curvature. The folds in Menetrier's syndrome are enlarged due to a glandular hyperplasia and are often concentrated in a plaque-like, fairly well delimited part of the stomach, especially the greater curvature of the body.

QUESTION 57

The correct answer to question 57 is (B). While ulceration is an essential component of the Zollinger-Ellison syndrome, multiple ulcerations also occur fairly frequently in gastrointestinal lymphoma. Hence, the presence of ulceration is not useful as a differential diagnostic sign. Lymphoma is *not* associated with gastric hypersecretion in contrast to the Zollinger-Ellison syndrome (see Figure 9-1, p. 56). Therefore, this is the most important differential diagnostic feature listed in this question. A retrogastric mass can occur in *both* diseases, in one case representing an unusually large non-beta islet cell tumor in the pancreas, in the other, retrogastric lymph node enlargement. Enlargement of the gastric mucosal folds also occurs in *both* diseases. In the case of lymphoma the large gastric folds are due to actual infiltration by the lymphomatous growth whereas in the Zollinger-Ellison syndrome they are usually inflammatory changes and hyperplasia of the parietal cell mass. The small bowel pattern can also be abnormal in *both* of these diseases due to either the enlargement of the folds and swelling associated with the Zollinger-Ellison syndrome or due to infiltration by neoplastic cells in the case of lymphoma.

QUESTION 58

The correct answer to question 58 is (A). As a matter of fact, all of the other answers are *true* statements about eosinophilic gastroenteritis and are, therefore, *incorrect* answers. In this disease gastric involvement is generally restricted to the *distal* portion of the stomach, and sometimes it may not involve the stomach at all. Granuloma with eosinophils is often a circumscribed polypoid lesion which can occur in almost any portion of the gastrointestinal tract and is not apparently related to eosinophilic granuloma as generally recognized in bone or lung.

DISCUSSION

Gastric lymphoma constitutes about 2 per cent of all neoplasms of the stomach. According to Sherrick *et al.*, three main types can be recognized, ulcerative (42 per cent), polypoid (47 per cent), and diffuse (11 per cent). An exact differential diagnosis from other neoplasms of the stomach may sometimes be difficult, if not impossible. In some cases, there may be a rather striking enlargement of retrogastric and other regional lymph nodes which may merge into the gastric involvement, owing to invasion of the stomach by the disease of the contiguous lymph nodes or extension of the gastric lesion to the immediately adjacent regional nodes. Enlargement of the spleen may be present, but is not necessary for the diagnosis.

One fairly characteristic roentgen sign separating the lymphomas from the carcinomas of the stomach is the relatively preserved *flexibility* of the stomach in lymphoma. This sign is well shown in the case illustrated here, being manifested by the obvious ability of the stomach to distend (Figure 25) and contract (Figure 26).

If the disease extends across the pylorus or involves other parts of the gastrointestinal tract in addition to the stomach, lymphoma is high on the list of possible diagnoses, since such multiple areas of disease are infrequent in carcinoma. Prognosis with appropriate therapy, especially radiation, is better than it is with carcinoma of the stomach.

Most lymphomas of the stomach are of the lymphocytic or the reticulum cell type. Hodgkin's disease is found much less frequently and almost without fail is associated with involvement in other parts of the body. However, retrogastric lymph node enlargement due to spread of Hodgkin's disease from other parts of the body is very common and the resulting gastric displacement is one of the indications for gastrointestinal roentgen examinations in patients with this disease. In view of the relative infrequency of primary involvement of the stomach in Hodgkin's disease, the possibility must be considered that a gastric lesion in the presence of Hodgkin's disease elsewhere is a *second* neoplasm. This may be due to decreased immunological resistance of the patient who has Hodgkin's disease. It appears that such a decrease in immunological competence may lead to an increased incidence of other neoplasms.

Pseudolymphoma, also called "gastric lymphoid hyperplasia" (a benign condition) enters the differential diagnosis of lymphoma of the stomach. On a single roentgen examination, this differential diagnosis is extremely difficult. The radiological findings, a prolonged clinical course, and the microscopic appearance together permit one to make a reasonably firm diagnosis. Even then it may sometimes be difficult, and occasionally what was thought to be a pseudolymphoma for several years eventually assumes the characteristics of a true malignant lymphoma. Pseudolymphomas are quite rare.

SUGGESTED READINGS

HYPERTROPHIC GASTRITIS

Berlin L: Gastritis: a medical dilemma. Am J Roentgenol *88:*627–636, 1962

ZOLLINGER-ELLISON SYNDROME

Zollinger RM, Grant GN: Ulcerogenic tumor of the pancreas. JAMA *190:*181–184, 1964
Also see bibliography on page 67

SUPERFICIAL SPREADING CARCINOMA

Bragg DG, Seaman WB, Lattes R: Roentgenologic and pathologic aspects cf superficial spreading carcinoma of the stomach. Am J Roentgenol *101:*437–443, 1967

GASTRIC LYMPHOMA

1. Bloch C: Roentgen features of Hodgkin's disease of the stomach. Am J Roentgenol *99:*175–181, 1967
2. Perez CA, Dorfman RF: Benign lymphoid hyperplasia of the stomach and duodenum. Radiology *87:*505–510, 1966
3. Sherrick DW, Hodgson JR, Dockerty MB: The roentgenologic diagnosis of primary gastric lymphoma. Radiology *84:*925–932, 1965

EOSINOPHILIC GASTROENTERITIS

1. Burhenne HJ, Carbone JV: Eosinophilic (allergic) gastroenteritis. Am J Roentgenol *96:*332–338, 1966
2. Kaplan SM, Goldstein F, Kowlessar OD: Eosinophilic gastroenteritis. Report of a case with malabsorption and protein-losing enteropathy. Gastroenterology *58:*540–545, 1970

MENETRIER'S DISEASE

1. Marshak RH, Wolf BS, Cohen N, Janowitz HD: Protein-losing disorders of the gastrointestinal tract: roentgen features. Radiology *77:*893–904, 1961
2. Reese DF, Hodgson JR, Dockerty MB: Giant hypertrophy of the gastric mucosa (Menetrier's disease): a correlation of the roentgenographic, pathologic and clinical findings. Am J Roentgenol *88:*619–626, 1962
3. Waldmann TA, Wochner RD, Strober W: The role of the gastrointestinal tract in plasma protein metabolism. Studies with ^{51}Cr-albumin. Am J Med *46:*275–285, 1969

CORRECT ANSWERS

Question 55-(D)
Question 56-(C)
Question 57-(B)
Question 58-(A)

NOTES

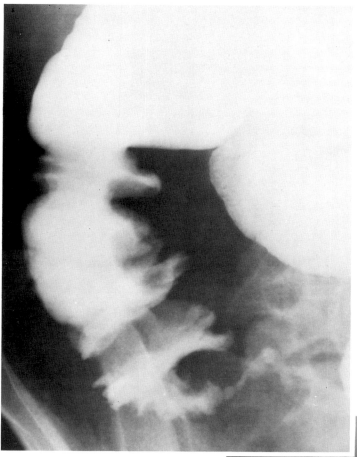

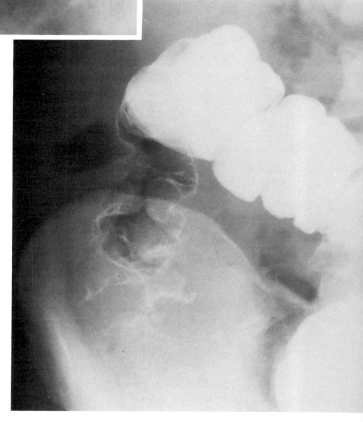

Figures 27 (*top*) *and 28* (*bottom*). This 45-year-old man has epigastric pain, diffuse abdominal tenderness, and voluntary muscle guarding. The filled (Figure 27) and postevacuation (Figure 28) roentgenograms of the cecum were made during a barium enema.

Questions 59 through 63

59. Which one of the following is the *MOST* likely diagnosis?

    (A) Lymphosarcoma
    (B) Tuberculosis
    (C) Carcinoma
    (D) Intramural hemorrhage
    (E) Granulomatous colitis

60. Which one of the following statements concerning primary lymphosarcoma of the colon is *LEAST* likely?

    (A) It occurs more commonly in the cecum than in other parts of the colon
    (B) It generally involves a longer segment than does carcinoma
    (C) It often produces widening of the lumen at the site of the lesion
    (D) It is common in children
    (E) It is less common than primary lymphosarcoma of the small intestine or stomach

61. Which one of the following is *MOST* likely to mimic ileocecal tuberculosis?

    (A) Granulomatous ileocolitis
    (B) Amebiasis
    (C) Ulcerative colitis
    (D) Carcinoma of the cecum
    (E) Lymphogranuloma venereum

62. The *MOST* suggestive roentgenographic manifestation of an intramural hemorrhage due to venous or arterial occlusion is

    (A) "thumbprinting"
    (B) multiple ulcerations
    (C) rigidity
    (D) spasm
    (E) fixation of the involved segment

63. Which one of the following statements concerning carcinoma of the cecum is *LEAST* likely?

   (A)   Iron deficiency anemia is a common manifestation
   (B)   Obstruction is an early manifestation
   (C)   Perforation is uncommon
   (D)   The lesion is most often polypoid
   (E)   It is less common than carcinoma of the rectum

Discussion

QUESTION 59

The correct answer to question 59 is (D). The several smoothly outlined sessile masses which indent the lumen of the cecum and ascending colon (*arrows* in Figures 28A and B) are highly suggestive of an intramural hemorrhage, especially when present in a portion of the colon or small intestine which is distensible (note the difference in caliber and shape of the cecum in Figures 27 and 28). Some of the smoothly defined indentations are due to the markedly enlarged mucosal folds which produce the so-called "transverse ridging" (*white arrows on left side* of Figure 28A), whereas other larger indentations (*arrows on right side* of Figure 28A) are due to intramural hemorrhages which result in the fusion of two or three contiguous folds to form each of the larger intraluminal polypoid masses. Although an intramural hemorrhage may encircle the cecum and ascending colon, the changes are usually first seen, and are most prominent, on the medial or mesenteric aspect. Since these marginal indentations resemble finger tips or thumb prints (Figure 28A, *medial arrows*), this appearance has been termed "thumbprinting". This sign is highly suggestive of intramural hemorrhage in the small or large intestine, particularly when seen on the mesenteric margin of the involved loop. The postevacuation view (Figure 28) shows a decrease in the caliber of the ascending colon as compared to the filled view (Figure 27), thus showing that there is definite pliability of the wall. On the postevacuation view of the contracted cecum, the polyp-like "thumbprints" (Figure 28B, *arrows*) indent both the medial and lateral aspects of the lumen which still contains enough air and barium to show the rather characteristic smooth surfaces of the indentations.

Localized primary lymphosarcoma could simulate an intramural hemorrhage, although the submucosal lymphomatous polypoid masses which indent the lumen are not usually as symmetrical and regular as those seen in this case. Furthermore, a large extrinsic mass is often associated with the mesenteric side of an intramural lymphomatous lesion if there is involvement of the adjacent lymph nodes. No evidence of such a mass is seen here. Also, it would be somewhat unusual for a lymphosarcoma to occur in a 45-year-old man, since it is more common in the older age groups. The patient whose roentgenograms are illustrated here had a rather acute clinical picture which would be unusual as the presenting feature of a lymphosarcoma, but quite typical of an intramural hemorrhage.

Ileocecal tuberculosis is almost always associated with cavitary pulmonary tuberculosis because it is apparently caused by the exposure of the ileal and cecal mucosa to large amounts of heavily infected sputum. It has now become a rare disease because of the marked improvement in the treatment of pulmonary tuberculosis. In ileocecal tuberculosis there is usually constant narrowing of the cecum due to the thickening of the wall by the firm granulomatous tissue, in contrast to the distensibility of the cecum in the case shown here. There are no pathognomonic roentgenographic signs of tuberculosis of the cecum and the only way to make a firm diagnosis is to verify microscopically the presence of caseation necrosis and isolate the tubercle bacillus from the diseased tissues. Therefore, tuberculosis of the cecum would not be the most likely diagnosis in this case.

QUESTION 60

The correct answer to question 60 is (D) because primary lymphosarcoma and other malignant neoplasms of the colon are extremely rare in children. In fact, it is difficult to find a documented case. All of the other possible responses listed are *true* statements about lymphosarcoma, and they are, therefore, *wrong* answers. Thus, lymphosarcoma *is* more common in the stomach and small intestine than in the colon, and it *is* more common in the cecum than in other parts of the colon. In general, lymphosarcomas tend to involve *longer* segments than do most carcinomas, although it is sometimes impossible to differentiate between the two diseases. One of the interesting features of lymphosarcoma is its tendency to produce *widening* of the lumen at the site of a large lesion, particularly those which involve the small intestine, in which case the portion of the mass adjacent to the lumen becomes necrotic, thus causing the "lumen" of the tumor to be wider than the normal lumen proximal or distal to the tumor. Conversely, this finding is not seen in carcinoma which usually causes narrowing of the lumen. This interesting phenomenon is called "aneurysmal dilatation" and

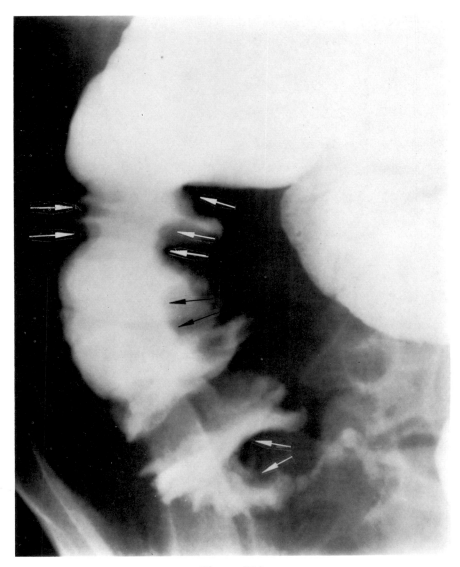

Figure 28A

probably accounts for the relatively low incidence of obstruction in cases of large lymphosarcomas, in contrast to the frequent presence of obstruction in the constricting annular carcinomas.

QUESTION 61

The correct answer to question 61 is (A). It is generally agreed that there are no roentgen findings which are diagnostic for ileocecal tuberculosis, and since all of the roentgen findings present in proven cases of ile-

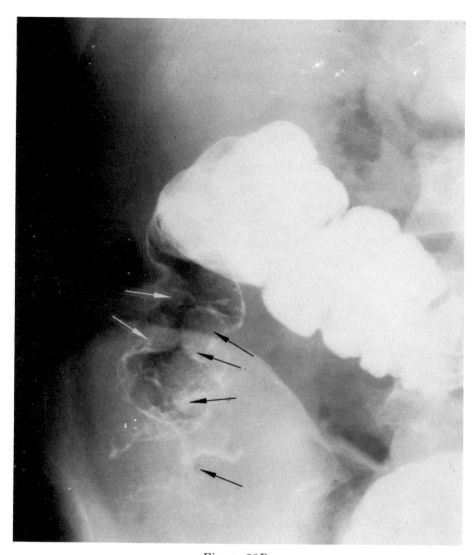

Figure 28B

ocecal tuberculosis *also* occur in the much more common granulomatous colitis (Crohn's disease), the latter condition is the one which would most likely mimic ileocecal tuberculosis. Both diseases produce *granulomatous* changes in the wall of the ileum and cecum.

Admittedly, in this case it would have been helpful to have seen the small intestine because of its frequent involvement in granulomatous disease, and if such involvement were present it would have favored the diagnosis of granulomatous ileocolitis. Unfortunately, the terminal ileum could not be filled during this examination. However, the "polypoid" lesions shown here

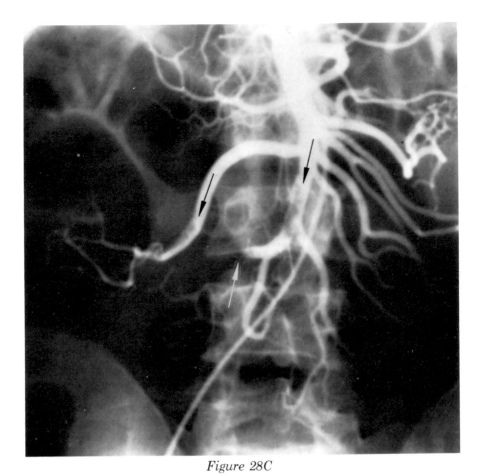

Figure 28C

NORMAL

GROSS APPEARANCE OF CECUM

MICROSCOPIC APPEARANCE OF CAPILLARIES

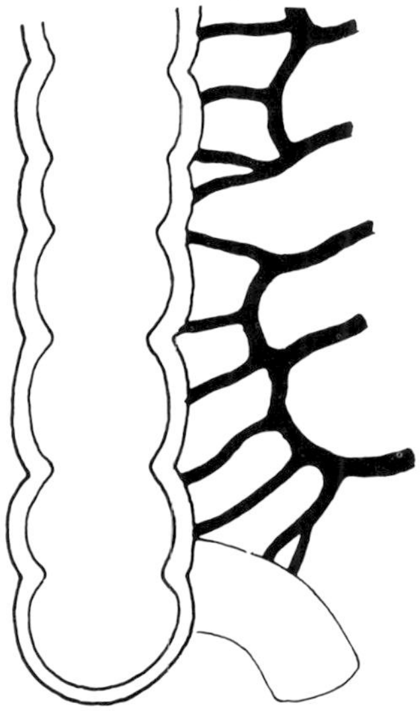

NORMAL

Figure 28D

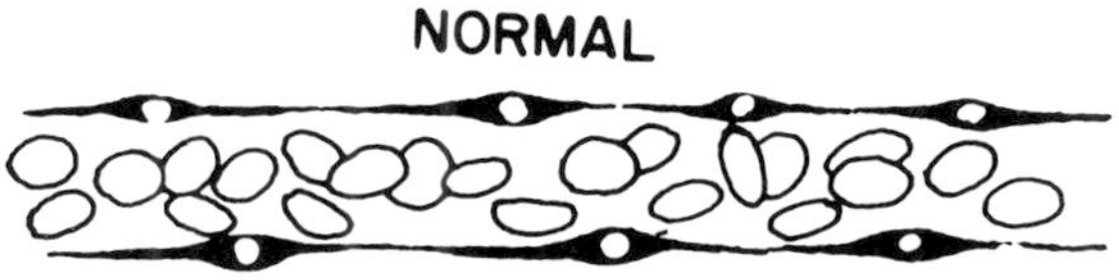

Figure 28E

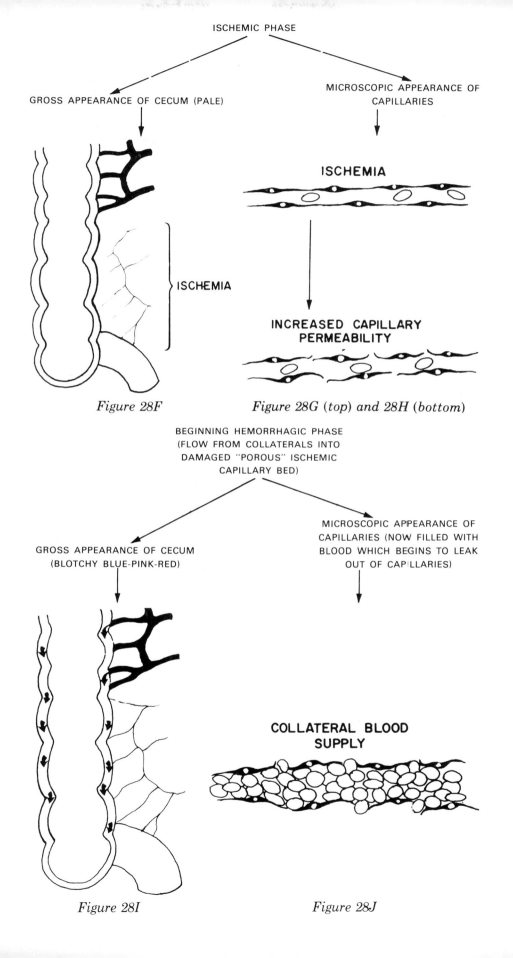

ISCHEMIC PHASE

GROSS APPEARANCE OF CECUM (PALE)

MICROSCOPIC APPEARANCE OF CAPILLARIES

ISCHEMIA

ISCHEMIA

INCREASED CAPILLARY PERMEABILITY

Figure 28F

Figure 28G (top) and 28H (bottom)

BEGINNING HEMORRHAGIC PHASE
(FLOW FROM COLLATERALS INTO
DAMAGED "POROUS" ISCHEMIC
CAPILLARY BED)

GROSS APPEARANCE OF CECUM
(BLOTCHY BLUE-PINK-RED)

MICROSCOPIC APPEARANCE OF
CAPILLARIES (NOW FILLED WITH
BLOOD WHICH BEGINS TO LEAK
OUT OF CAPILLARIES)

COLLATERAL BLOOD
SUPPLY

Figure 28I

Figure 28J

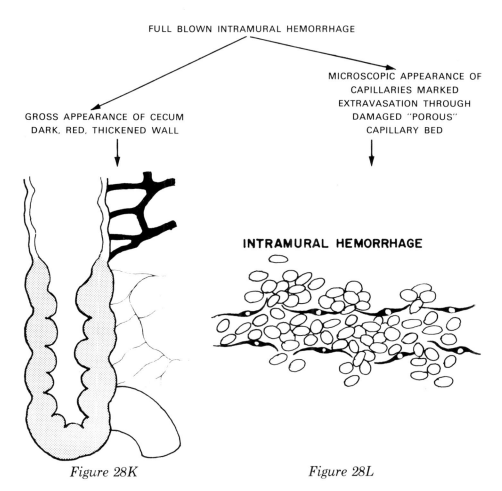

FULL BLOWN INTRAMURAL HEMORRHAGE

GROSS APPEARANCE OF CECUM
DARK, RED, THICKENED WALL

MICROSCOPIC APPEARANCE OF
CAPILLARIES MARKED
EXTRAVASATION THROUGH
DAMAGED "POROUS"
CAPILLARY BED

INTRAMURAL HEMORRHAGE

Figure 28K   *Figure 28L*

are somewhat larger, rounder, smoother, and more localized on the mesenteric side of the bowel than the "cobblestones" or "pseudopolyps" seen
in most cases of granulomatous colitis. The absence of longitudinal or transverse ulcers also militates somewhat against granulomatous colitis. Furthermore, granulomatous colitis is not usually localized to such a short segment
of the colon, and the thickened rigid walls of a granulomatous lesion do not
usually permit as much change in caliber of the lumen as shown in the case
presented here.

Amebiasis and ulcerative colitis do not ordinarily produce the large polypoid type of lesions and marked thickening of the bowel wall which
characterize the granulomatous diseases and would, therefore, not be likely
to mimic ileocecal tuberculosis. It would also be unusual for ulcerative
colitis to be so localized, particularly in the cecum, since it characteristically involves the left side of the colon. Since carcinoma of the cecum does
not ordinarily involve the ileum, it would not be likely to mimic ileocecal

tuberculosis. Lymphogranuloma venereum involves the distal end of the colon contiguous to the diseased pelvic portion of the genitourinary tract, and ordinarily does not involve the cecum, ileum, or other parts of the digestive tract which lie above the pelvis.

Since the lesion shown here involves the entire circumference of the colon, it could be misinterpreted as an annular carcinoma. However, an annular carcinoma is almost always characterized by an *abrupt* transition between the carcinoma and the adjacent normal colon. We do not see such an appearance here. Furthermore, a carcinoma usually has an *irregular fuzzy* surface due to mucosal destruction and nodularity, thus differing from the smooth surfaces of the multiple rounded intramural masses seen here. Also, an annular carcinoma as large as the lesion illustrated here would be so *rigid* that it would virtually preclude the noticeable change in caliber of the lumen seen in this case. Therefore, the diagnosis of an annular carcinoma is not justified.

QUESTION 62

The answer to question 62 is (A). Of all the possible answers listed, "thumbprinting" is the only one which is suggestive of venous or arterial occlusion. It must be emphasized that "thumbprinting" is merely a term used to describe the marginal indentations produced by the submucosal hemorrhages which occur in the bowel wall, and it must be kept in mind that marginal indentations of the lumen can occur in diseases which produce polypoid masses or considerable enlargement of the mucosal folds. However, other lesions, such as multiple colon polyps, lymphosarcomas (see Figures 31, 32, 33 and 34, pp. 166 and 168), or granulomatous disease, are not characterized by such smoothly defined symmetrical "thumbprints" as those seen in this case.

QUESTION 63

The correct answer to question 63 is (B) because obstruction is *not* an early manifestation of *carcinoma* of the cecum. The cecum usually has the widest lumen of the entire colon and obstruction does not occur until late in the cource of the disease at a time when the carcinoma has become quite large. Cecal carcinomas are more frequently polypoid than annular, and this is a plausible reason for the late development of obstruction. All of the other possible responses listed are *correct* statements about carcinoma of the cecum, and are, therefore, *wrong* responses to this question.

DISCUSSION

When the roentgen findings seen here are associated with acute abdominal distress in a patient who has heart disease, hemorrhagic disease, a hypercoagulability state, or peripheral vascular disease, they should strongly suggest an intramural hemorrhage due to a vascular occlusion or a hemorrhagic diathesis. In order to be absolutely certain about the diagnosis in this case, superior mesenteric arteriography was performed (Figure 28C). There is an occlusion of of the ileocolic artery about 1 cm. distal to its origin (*white arrow*) and there are several radiolucent intraluminal masses (*two black arrows*) due to thrombi or emboli in the right colic artery and in the main trunk of the superior mesenteric artery distal to the origin of the right colic artery. Such selective superior mesenteric arteriographic studies, although not always necessary, are quite helpful when available, since they not only demonstrate the occluded vessels, but also can help determine the etiology of the obstruction and identify additional unsuspected thrombi or emboli, as was true in this case. Such studies are of great value if surgical intervention becomes necessary, as it sometimes does.

This patient was treated with anticoagulants, following which he made a complete recovery. The clinical importance of recognizing intramural hemorrhages is related to the fact that most of them will resolve *without* operative treatment unless they are so extensive that ischemic necrosis ensues. Many of these lesions will regress spontaneously and the bowel will revert to a normal roentgenological appearance if good collateral circulation is established. If ischemia results only in a moderate amount of tissue necrosis in a short segment of bowel, a stricture may result. On the other hand, if *extensive* necrosis occurs due to occlusive disease of multiple vessels, or due to the occlusion of a major vessel such as the main trunk of the superior mesenteric artery, an operation may become necessary in order to avoid a fatal outcome. In such cases the unfavorable clinical response of the patient to supportive measures is usually clearly indicated by a rapidly rising polymorphonuclear leukocytosis, unrelenting abdominal pain, and shock.

It is important to keep in mind that treatment with anticoagulants can result in *further intramural hemorrhage*. Thus, not only is immediate operation unnecessary in most cases, due to the reversible nature of the ischemia, but treatment with anticoagulants must be judiciously employed and carefully controlled to avoid exaggeration of the intramural bleeding.

The sequence of events (Figures 28D through L) in the formation of a submucosal hemorrhage following a vascular occlusion is related to the severe damage which occurs in the ischemic capillary bed *distal* to the occlusion. The endothelial cells in the damaged capillary bed can no longer adhere to one another (Figure 28H) so that the blood which later flows into the damaged capillary bed *via* the collateral circulation (Figures 28I and J) will flow through the porous endothelial "sieve" (Figure 28L) into the interstitial areas of the bowel to form an intramural hematoma (Figure 28K) as shown on the roentgenographic illustrations in this case (Figures 27 and 28). The tumor-like masses may sometimes become so large that their encroachment upon the lumen may be great enough to occlude it.

The intramural hemorrhages which occur in patients with idiopathic thrombocytopenic purpura and hemophilia are related to other abnormalities rather than to the ischemia which results from occlusive vascular disease. However, the intramural hemorrhages which occur in these hematological diseases have the *same* roentgen appearance as those which occur subsequent to intravascular occlusions.

In summary, it should be emphasized that the radiologist who correctly suspects or makes the diagnosis of an intramural hemorrhage can make a significant contribution to the proper management of these patients. Although the diagnosis can be strongly suspected if the patient has an associated disease which is etiologically related to the formation of an intramural hemorrhage, it becomes virtually certain when the barium study shows the characteristic "thumbprinting", transverse ridging, and pliability of a localized segment of the bowel wall. As the late Merrill Sosman was accustomed to emphasize: "We see what we look for, and we recognize what we know."

SUGGESTED READINGS

INTRAMURAL HEMORRHAGE

1. Boley SJ, Schwartz S, Lash J, Sternhill V: Reversible vascular occlusion of the colon. Surg Gynecol & Obstet *116:*53–60, 1963
2. Dunbar JD, Nelson SW: Nonangiographic manifestations of intestinal vascular disease. Am J Roentgenol *99:*127–135, 1967
3. Engelhardt JE, Jacobson G: Infarction of the colon demonstrated by barium enema. Radiology *67:*573–575, 1956
4. Marshak RH, Lindner AE: Vascular diseases of the small bowel and colon. In AR Margulis, HJ Burhenne: *Alimentary Tract Roentgenology*, Chap 47. CV Mosby Co, St. Louis, 1967
5. Schwartz S, Boley SJ, Robinson K, Krieger H, Schultz L, Allen AC: Roentgenologic features of vascular disorders of the intestines. Radiol Clin North Am *2:*71–87, 1964

LYMPHOSARCOMA

1. Dreyfuss JR, Janower ML: The colon. In LL Robbins (ed): *Golden's Diagnostic Radiology, Section 5: Digestive Tract*, pp 890–900. Williams & Wilkins Co, Baltimore, 1969
2. Woodruff JH Jr, Skorneck AB: Malignant lymphoma of the colon and rectum: roentgen diagnosis. California Med *96:*181–183, 1962

3. Wychulis AR, Beahrs OH, Woolner LB: Malignant lymphoma of the colon: a study of 69 cases. Arch Surg *93:*215–225, 1966

ILEOCECAL TUBERCULOSIS *VERSUS* GRANULOMATOUS COLITIS

1. Brombart M, Massion J: Radiologic differences between ileocecal tuberculosis and Crohn's disease. I. Diagnosis of ileocecal tuberculosis. Am J Digestive Dis NS *6:*589–603, 1961
2. Dreyfus JR, Janower ML: The colon. In LL Robbins (ed): *Golden's Diagnostic Radiology, Section 5: Digestive Tract*, pp 869–870. Williams & Wilkins Co, Baltimore, 1969
3. Paustian FF: Tuberculosis of the intestines. In HL Bockus: *Gastroenterology, Vol II*, 2nd ed, pp 311–334. WB Saunders Co, Philadelphia, 1964

CARCINOMA OF CECUM

Dreyfuss JR, Janower ML: The colon. In LL Robbins (ed): *Golden's Diagnostic Radiology, Section 5: Digestive Tract*, pp 886–887. Williams & Wilkins Co, Baltimore, 1969

LYMPHOGRANULOMA VENEREUM

1. Buckstein J: *The Digestive Tract in Roentgenology, Vol II*, 2nd ed, Chap 54. JB Lippincott Co, Philadelphia, 1953
2. Pessel JF: Lymphogranuloma venereum. In HL Bockus: *Gastroenterology, Vol II*, 2nd ed, Chap 76. WB Saunders Co, Philadelphia, 1964

CORRECT ANSWERS

Question 59-(D)
Question 60-(D)
Question 61-(A)
Question 62-(A)
Question 63-(B)

NOTES

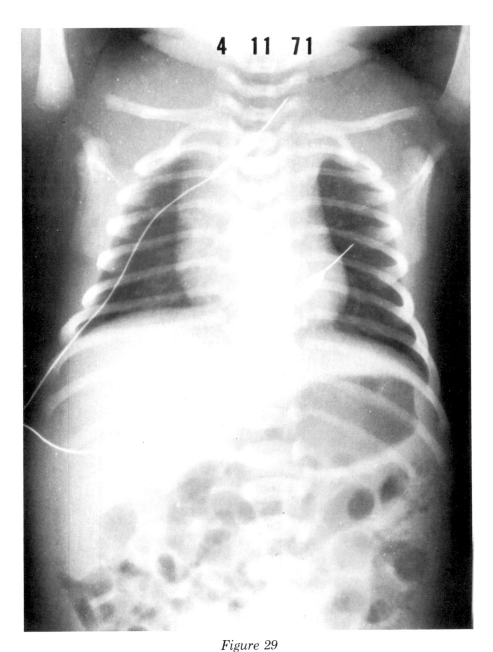

Figure 29

Figures 29 and 30. This premature girl was examined 48 hours after birth because of vomiting and abdominal distention. Roentgenograms of the patient in the supine position were taken at the time of examination (Figure 29) and after her condition had worsened (Figure 30).

Questions 64 through 68

64. Which one of the following is the *MOST* likely diagnosis?

   (A)   Meconium peritonitis
   (B)   Meconium ileus
   (C)   Necrotizing enterocolitis
   (D)   Aganglionosis
   (E)   "Meconium plug" syndrome

65. Meconium peritonitis is *MOST* frequently associated with which one of the following?

   (A)   Pneumoperitoneum
   (B)   Malrotation
   (C)   Mucoviscidosis
   (D)   Small bowel atresia
   (E)   Prematurity

66. Meconium ileus is associated with which one of the following conditions?

   (A)   Meconium peritonitis
   (B)   Small bowel atresia
   (C)   Fibrocystic disease
   (D)   Biliary atresia
   (E)   Gas in the wall of the gut

67. Which one of the following is *LEAST* characteristic of necrotizing enterocolitis?

   (A)   Intramural gas
   (B)   Perforation
   (C)   Prematurity
   (D)   Severe diarrhea
   (E)   Respiratory distress

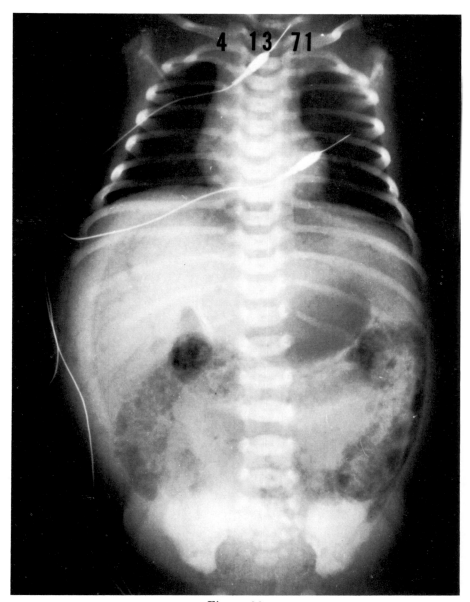

Figure 30

68. Which one of the following statements concerning congenital aganglionosis of the colon is *INCORRECT*?

(A) The aganglionic segment is not dilated

(B) It is limited to the rectum and a contiguous portion of the sigmoid in most patients

(C) It is not related to congenital microcolon

(D) Excessive retention of barium in the colon for more than 24—48 hours after barium enema is an early finding in young infants

(E) It may involve the entire colon

Discussion

QUESTION 64

The correct answer to question 64 is (C), this being a typical example of necrotizing enterocolitis of the newborn. The illustration of the film dated 4-11-71 (Figure 29) shows no abnormal findings in the chest or abdomen. However, on the photograph of the film dated 4-13-71 (Figure 30) there are several important radiological findings which indicate the presence of a significant and dangerous condition which threatens the infant's life. In the newborn it is normally difficult, if not impossible, to differentiate small bowel and colon gas, and this is true on the first illustration (Figure 29). However, 2 days later (Figure 30) the colon can be recognized because of its distention by what, at first glance, *appears* to be a mixture of solid fecal material and gas. It is unusual for the colon of a newborn infant to be so clearly depicted on plain roentgenograms. It is also abnormal for such an infant's colon to be filled with what appears to be the solid adult-type of fecal material mixed with gas, since infant stools are usually quite liquid in consistency.

How, then, does one explain these findings? First, the somewhat "bubbly" appearance of the colon is not due to the adult-type of formed stools but is due to a combination of findings which includes intraluminal blood, sloughed colonic mucosa, intraluminal gas, and some fecal material. One of the reasons the colon is so well outlined is that there is *gas* in the wall, which is particularly well seen on the lateral margin of the descending colon (*white arrows* in Figure 30A). In necrotizing enterocolitis there is often a varying amount of gas in the wall of the colon, and multiple small localized collections which are seen *en face* are superimposed over the gas-containing colonic contents, so as to cast additional shadows which contribute to the "bubbly" appearance. Such an appearance of the colon is virtually diagnostic of necrotizing enterocolitis.

On seeing this condition, one looks for several additional corroborative findings usually associated with it. First, one looks for gas in the portal venous system in the liver. Indeed, such gas collections are clearly seen (Figure 30A, *small black oblique arrows*). This is due to the passage of interstitial gas from the wall of the colon into the damaged capillary bed and, hence, into the portal venous system of the liver. Another well known complication of necrotizing enterocolitis is the tendency for the colon to perforate and cause pneumoperitoneum. This is often manifested, as it is here, by a faint oval radiolucency which is superimposed over the entire abdomen. This is particularly well shown in the right flank area where the intraperitoneal gas can be seen at its interface (*large black arrows*, Figure 30A) with the parietal peritoneum of the lateral part of the abdominal wall. This vague radiolucency is best appreciated by comparing the abnormal radiolucency in the liver region (Figure 30) with the same area (Figure 29) on which the liver area has the normal homogeneous water density. In fact, there is an increased radiolucency of the entire abdomen (Figure 30) as compared to the normal appearance (Figure 29). This oval radiolucency of the abdomen has been termed the "football sign" and is due to the large amount of free gas in the uppermost (anterior) portion of the peritoneal cavity where it will accumulate when a patient lies in the supine position during the roentgen examination, as was true in this case. One can further corroborate the presence of pneumoperitoneum on such a supine roentgenogram by looking for the shadow of the falciform ligament which is outlined only when there is gas on both sides of it. Then it appears as a curvilinear water-density shadow to the right of the spine (Figure 30A, *small horizontal arrows*) since the patient whose films are illustrated here had a large pneumoperitoneum and was lying in the supine position when the roentgenograms were made.

Meconium peritonitis is a condition which develops *in utero* during fetal life and is generally believed due to a perforation of the small intestine proximal to a high-grade or complete obstruction. It is believed that such a perforation on the proximal high-pressure side of an obstructing lesion allows meconium to pass into the peritoneum where it produces an inflammatory reaction (peritonitis) which, in time, results in calcifications which are usually clearly recognizable at birth. These calcifications are often only small flecks scattered throughout the abdomen, although there may sometimes be larger conglomerates of calcium along the inferior surface of the liver or concentrated in the flanks. Sometimes they occur on the serosa of the bowel wall and, thus, are often curvilinear and parallel if both walls of one loop of bowel are involved. The roentgen findings of mechanical ileus are often seen in infants with calcifications due to meconium peritonitis. This is because the perforations which led to the meconium peritonitis may have healed, whereas the obstructing lesion, such as ileal atresia or inspissated meconium remains and causes the radiological picture of mechanical ileus on plain roentgenograms following birth. Since the calcifications ordinarily associated with meconium peritonitis are not seen here, this would certainly not be the most likely diagnosis.

The absence of roentgenographic findings of small bowel distention (Figure 30) would militate strongly against meconium ileus, in which condition there are usually numerous dilated loops of small bowel which are filled with fluid and gas. Since the fluid in the distended loops of small bowel is sometimes rather thick and viscous in patients with meconium ileus, the gas collections may sometimes appear somewhat "bubbly" or "frothy" on plain films. However, it is usually difficult to differentiate the dilated loops of small bowel and colon in meconium ileus, in contrast to the easily recognized distended colon in the case presented here. In fact, there is relatively little recognizable small bowel gas, but a moderate amount of gas is identifiable in the stomach immediately above the transverse colon. Thus, on the roentgenograms illustrated here, there are none of the findings of meconium ileus.

Although aganglionosis does not usually manifest itself during the first few days of life, it should be considered whenever there is generalized distention manifested by multiple air- and fluid-filled loops of bowel. In the case presented here, the only recognizable distended organ is the *colon*; and the rather classical appearance of the "bubbly" fecal material, the intramural gas, the pneumoperitoneum, and gas in the portal venous system clearly favor necrotizing enterocolitis rather than aganglionosis. Although patients with aganglionosis can, indeed, develop necrotizing enterocolitis as a complication, it is doubtful that the aganglionosis would have reached such a serious stage as to cause perforation this soon after birth. Thus, uncomplicated aganglionosis would not be the most likely diagnosis.

The "meconium plug" syndrome is seen in newborn infants, but the plugs of meconium in the left side of the colon usually result in a relatively normal or smaller-than-normal caliber distal to the plug (or plugs) and distention of the colon with fluid and gas proximal to the obstruction. Sometimes clumps of water-density meconium can be seen in the gas-filled colon proximal to the obstruction. Conversely, in the case shown here, virtually the entire colon is filled with what appears to be "feces-like" material which has the unusual "bubbly" appearance noted earlier in the discussion. The "meco-

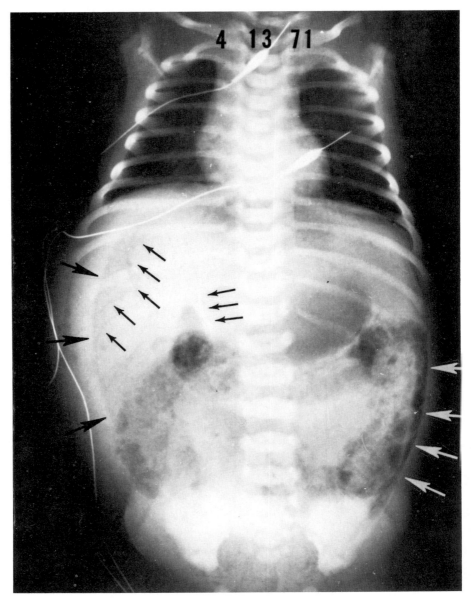

Figure 30A

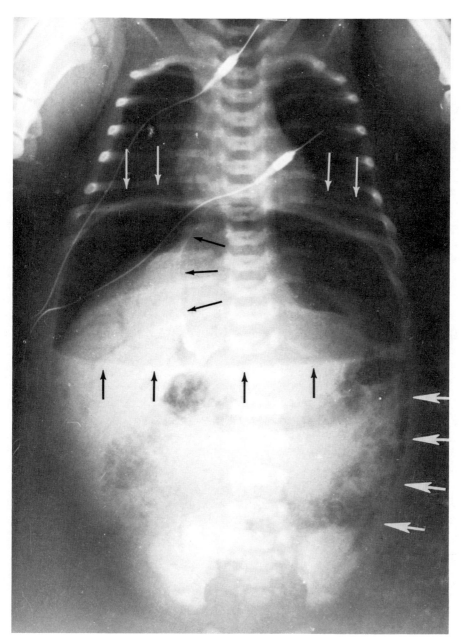

Figure 30B

nium plug" syndrome is usually relieved by enemas, and usually does not result in necrotizing colitis with pneumoperitoneum and gas in the portal venous system.

QUESTION 65

The answer to question 65 is (D). Meconium peritonitis is almost always associated with small bowel atresia which causes *complete obstruction*. Thus, an infant with meconium peritonitis would not be expected to have gas in the colon, in contrast to the case shown here. Furthermore, abdominal calcifications are often present in meconium peritonitis, whereas none is seen in the case presented here. A barium enema study in infants with meconium peritonitis will often show spectacular evidence of a microcolon ("unused colon") and the reflux of barium into the terminal ileum may show the point of obstruction to the retrograde flow if the obstruction is due to ileal atresia. However, such a retrograde barium study of the ileum is not usually necessary in patients with a picture of an unused colon and meconium peritonitis (peritoneal calcifications). Meconium peritonitis is not ordinarily associated with pneumoperitoneum since the perforation through which meconium entered the peritoneum is usually not evident at birth. Presumably most of these perforations heal *in utero*. Meconium peritonitis has no causal relationship to malrotation of the colon. Meconium *ileus* is usually seen in patients with mucoviscidosis (fibrocystic disease), whereas most cases of meconium *peritonitis* are associated with complete obstructions due to ileal atresia rather than the partial obstructions caused by the viscid meconium which is found in patients with mucoviscidosis (fibrocystic disease). Although meconium ileus may occasionally be seen in premature infants, there is apparently no etiologic relationship between the two.

QUESTION 66

The correct answer to question 66 is (C) because meconium ileus is frequently associated with fibrocystic disease of the pancreas (mucoviscidosis). In this disease the meconium is much more viscid than normal due to the deficiency in pancreatic secretions caused by congenital stenosis of the pancreatic duct system or disease of the pancreatic acini. As a result, the thick and sticky meconium cannot be readily propelled through the small intestine of the fetus. Although meconium peritonitis is most frequently associated with small bowel atresia, it is occasionally seen in infants with meconium ileus. Meconium ileus does not occur with biliary atresia since the presence of bile apparently has no influence on the consistency of the meconium. Meconium ileus is not associated with gas in the wall of the colon.

QUESTION 67

Whereas intramural gas, pneumoperitoneum (perforation), and respiratory distress in a premature infant *are* characteristic of necrotizing enterocolitis, *severe* diarrhea is *not common*. Since severe diarrhea is the least characteristic of the list of possible responses, **the correct answer to question 67 is (D).** Although there may be a few loose blood-streaked stools in about one half of the infants who have necrotizing enterocolitis, severe diarrhea is surprisingly infrequent. Babies who develop this condition are usually born prematurely and may seem otherwise healthy during the first 48 to 72 hours of life, during which respiration may be normal and the infant may feed normally. However, the infant then begins to vomit bile-tinged material, develops mild-to-severe abdominal distention and respiratory distress, the course usually being progressively downhill unless vigorous therapeutic measures are instituted.

QUESTION 68

The answer to question 68 is (C) since all of the other possible responses listed are *correct* statements about aganglionosis. Congenital aganglionosis *is* one of the causes of "congenital microcolon" which is only a descriptive term applying to the small colon associated with congenital diseases. Microcolon is frequently associated with ileal atresia, in which case it is small because it is *unused*. It is not usually seen in patients with congenital aganglionosis unless the aganglionosis involves the *entire* colon, in which case the colon may appear somewhat small in caliber ("microcolon") in comparison to the dilated small bowel. The lack of normal peristaltic activity in the aganglionic "microcolon" produces what might be termed a physiological obstruction of the small intestine rather than a mechanical one.

DISCUSSION

Necrotizing enterocolitis is a serious disease at any age, but it is particularly life-threatening in a newborn infant, and especially those born prematurely. The disease often occurs in premature infants who have no other complicating etiological conditions. It may also occur in full-term infants in association with such potentially causative factors as intestinal obstruction, as often occurs in the common form of aganglionosis which involves the *distal* portion of the colon. Necrotizing enterocolitis may rarely occur in debilitated infants with intestinal atresia, stenosis, or meconium ileus. In fatal cases the deterioration is usually progressive and rapid, with spells of apnea, jaundice, shock, and death. Infants with severe distention are sometimes surgically explored, either for the perforation indicated by the pneumoperitoneum found on roentgen examination, or because aganglionic megacolon is suspected.

Although necrotizing enterocolitis may occasionally simulate neonatal aganglionosis clinically, the onset of the abdominal distention and vomiting associated with the latter condition usually does not begin until some time between the third and fifth days of life; i.e., somewhat later than necrotizing enterocolitis which so frequently has its onset between 48 and 72 hours after birth. The intramural gas seen in the colon of patients with necrotizing enterocolitis should not be confused with "pneumatosis coli" of the adult (see Figure 7, p. 42) which is a benign form of intramural gas usually occurring on the left side of the colon. The gas in the wall of the colon in necrotizing enterocolitis is probably related to necrosis of the mucosa and subsequent passage of intraluminal gas into the wall of the colon. This situation is probably also complicated by the presence of intraluminal gas-forming organisms which penetrate the diseased mucosa to form intramural gas. Regardless of the exact way in which gas reaches the interstices of the bowel wall, it often finds its way into the damaged capillary bed and reaches the intrahepatic branches of the portal vein where it can be identified on roentgenograms, as shown here. The latter finding is an ominous sign and death often (but not always) occurs within 24 hours unless prompt and vigorous therapy is instituted. Pneumoperitoneum is usually a late occurrence after extensive necrosis results in perforation of the bowel wall. Once pneumoperitoneum occurs the prognosis is grave. In fact, the patient whose films are illustrated here expired a few hours after the examination of 4–13–71 was made. However, more recent studies have shown that about 50 per cent of newborn infants with necrotizing enterocolitis can be saved with vigorous therapy.

Necrotizing enterocolitis commonly involves the ileum and right colon, but total gut involvement may occur. Variable mucosal destruction is present and a dirty brown pseudomembrane often covers the denuded areas. The bowel wall is often thickened and friable in the areas of involvement and multiple perforations may be present. Gross and microscopic evidence of intramural gas is often present in the submucosa, subserosa, and the pseudomembrane.

The typical roentgenologic findings on plain films and the clinical picture of necrotizing enterocolitis preclude the need for a barium enema. Indeed, a barium enema might be somewhat hazardous in view of the friable consistency of the colon. If a barium study of the colon is done, it may show findings which mimic those cases of aganglionic megacolon in which the aganglionic segment is located in the distal part of the colon. In such cases of aganglionic megacolon there is dilatation of the normal colon with stasis proximal to the aganglionic segment. This dilated portion of the colon may thus simulate the dilatation and stasis which occur in necrotizing enterocolitis.

The etiology of necrotizing enterocolitis is not known. It is possible that the immunological mechanisms are not yet normally developed in these infants, particularly the premature ones. Although there is a high incidence of maternal and fetal infection, no specific organism can be implicated. Similarly, the cause of the intramural gas collections is unknown, although bacteriogenic gas formed in the infected colon wall and the passage of intraluminal gas through necrotic breaks in the mucosa are probably the factors which are most commonly involved. The suggested mechanisms associated in many cases of pneumatosis cystoides intestinalis in adults (see discussion on pp. 48–51) are not involved in the development of necrotizing enterocolitis.

With prompt diagnosis, vigorous supportive medical care, and operative removal of necrotic bowel, recovery is possible in many cases. Residual changes in the colon may be seen in patients who recover without resection, such changes consisting of nodular submucosal infiltrates resembling benign lymphoid hyperplasia. In some cases there may be stricture formation as a result of mucosal sloughing.

An upright or decubitus roentgenogram of the abdomen will usually clarify doubtful cases of pneumoperitoneum. Such a roentgenogram should always be obtained in suspected cases of necrotizing enterocolitis because of the frequent presence of perforation in this condition. An illustration of the roentgenogram made with the patient in the upright position (Figure 30B) shows the huge pneumoperitoneum beneath both leaves of the diaphragm (*upper vertical arrows*). Also note the faintly seen falciform ligament (*horizontal black arrows*) and the confirmatory evidence of gas in the hepatic veins. Also note that the configuration of the colon gas on the roentgenogram made in the upright position *does not change* when compared to its appearance in the supine position. Particularly note that the linear gas collection in the left flank (*horizontal white arrows*, Figures 30A and B) remains unchanged, thus confirming its location in the wall of the colon. There are no recognizable intraluminal gas-fluid levels, and, thus, no identifiable small bowel loops, in contrast to the clearly outlined colon. The long single intraperitoneal gas-fluid level (*lower vertical arrows*) indicates peritonitis as a result of the perforation.

SUGGESTED READINGS

MECONIUM PERITONITIS

1. Harris JH, DeMuth WE Jr, Harris JH Jr: Meconium peritonitis: report of a case in which the diagnostic roentgen signs were found ante partum. Am J Roentgenol 76:555–557, 1956

2. Kasmersky CT, Howard WHR: The significance of intra-abdominal calcifications in the newborn infant. Am J Roentgenol 68:395–398, 1952
3. Neuhauser EBD: Roentgen diagnosis of fetal meconium peritonitis. Am J Roentgenol 51:421–425, 1944

MECONIUM ILEUS

1. Donnison AB, Shwachman H, Gross RE: A review of 164 children with meconium ileus seen at the Children's Hospital Medical Center, Boston. Pediatrics 37:833–850, 1966
2. Herson RE: Meconium ileus. Radiology 68:568–571, 1957
3. Leonidas, J, Berdon WE, Baker DH, Santulli TV: Meconium ileus and its complications. Am J Roentgenol 108:598–609, 1970
4. Wagget J: Nonoperative treatment of meconium ileus by Gastrografin enema. J Pediat 77:407, 1970
5. White H: Meconium ileus: new roentgen sign. Radiology 66:567–571, 1956

NECROTIZING ENTEROCOLITIS

1. Berdon WE, Grossman H, Baker DH, Mizrahi A, Barlow O, Blanc WA: Necrotizing enterocolitis in the premature infant. Radiology 83:879–887, 1964
2. Cohn R, Sunshine R, deVries P: Necrotizing enterocolitis in the newborn infant. Am J Surg 124:165–168, 1972
3. Rabinowitz JG, Wolf BS, Feller MR, Krasna I: Colonic changes following necrotizing enterocolitis in the newborn. Am J Roentgenol 103:359–364, 1963
4. Stevenson JK, Graham CB, Oliver TK, Goldenberg VE: Neonatal necrotizing enterocolitis: a report of twenty-one cases with fourteen survivors. Am J Surg 118:260–272, 1969.

AGANGLIONOSIS

1. Berdon WE, Baker DH: The roentgenographic diagnosis of Hirschsprung's disease in infancy. Am J Roentgenol 93:432–446, 1965
2. Berdon WE, Koontz P, Baker DH: Diagnosis of colonic and terminal ileal aganglionosis. Am J Roentgenol 91:680–689, 1964
3. Hiatt RB: The pathologic physiology of congenital megacolon. Ann Surg 133:313, 1951
4. Hope JW, Borns PF, Berg PK: Radiologic manifestations of Hirschsprung's disease in infancy. Am J Roentgenol 95:217–229, 1965
5. Swenson O, Davidson FJ: Similarities in mechanical obstruction and aganglionic megacolon in the newborn infant. New England J Med 262:46, 1960

"MECONIUM PLUG" SYNDROME

1. Clatworthy HW Jr, Howard WHR, Lloyd J: The meconium plug syndrome. Surgery 39:131–142, 1956
2. Ellis DG, Clatworthy HW Jr: Meconium plug syndrome revisited. J Pediat Surg 1:54–61, 1966
3. Mikity VG, Hodgman JE, Paciulli J: Meconium blockage syndrome. Radiology 88:740–744, 1967

PNEUMOPERITONEUM IN THE NEWBORN

1. Mestel AL, Trusler GA, Humphreys RP: Pneumoperitoneum in the newborn. Canadian M A J 95:201–204, 1966

2. Miller RE: Perforated viscus in infants: a new roentgen sign. Radiology *74:*65–67, 1960

3. Waldhausen JA, Herendeen T, King H: Necrotizing colitis of the newborn: common cause of perforation of the colon. Surgery *54:*365–372, 1963

4. Wolf JN, Evans WA: Gas in the portal veins of the liver in infants. Am J Roentgenol *74:*486–489, 1955

MALROTATION

1. Berdon WE, Baker HD, Bull S, Santulli TV: Midgut malrotation and volvulus. Radiology *96:*375–383, 1970

2. Findlay CW, Humphreys GH II: Congenital anomalies of intestinal rotation in the adult. Surg Gynecol & Obstet *103:*417, 1958

3. McIntosh R, Donovan EJ: Disturbances of rotation of the intestinal tract. Am J Dis Child *57:*116, 1939

CYSTIC FIBROSIS (MUCOVISCIDOSIS)

1. Bruwer A, Hodgson JR: Intestinal obstruction in fibrocystic disease of the pancreas. Am J Roentgenol *69:*14–21, 1953

2. Elian E: Usefulness of the sweat electrolyte test in differential diagnosis. New England J Med *264:*18, 1961

3. Grossman H, Berdon WE, Baker DH: Gastrointestinal findings in cystic fibrosis. Am J Roentgenol *97:*227–238, 1966

4. Neuhauser EBD: Roentgen changes associated with pancreatic insufficiency in early life. Radiology *46:*319–328, 1946

SMALL BOWEL ATRESIA

1. Bernstein J, Vawter G, Harris GB, Young V, Hillman LS: The occurrence of intestinal atresia in the newborn with meconium ileus: pathogenesis of an acquired anomaly. Am J Dis Child *99:*804–818, 1960

2. Steinfeld JR, Harrison RB: Extensive intramural intestinal calcification in a newborn with intestinal atresia. Case report. Radiology *107:*405–406, 1973

BILIARY ATRESIA

Farber S: Relation of pancreatic achylia to meconium ileus. J Pediat *24:*387–392, 1944

CONGENITAL MICROCOLON

1. Berdon WE, Baker DH, Santulli TV, Amoury RA, Blanc WA: Microcolon in newborn infants with intestinal obstruction. Radiology *90:*878–885, 1968

2. Sane SM, Girdany BR: Total aganglionosis coli. Clinical and roentgenographic manifestations. Radiology *107:*397–404, 1973

3. Zimmer, J: Microcolon with report of two cases. Acta Radiol *29:*228–236, 1948

CORRECT ANSWERS

Question 64-(C)
Question 65-(D)
Question 66-(C)
Question 67-(D)
Question 68-(C)

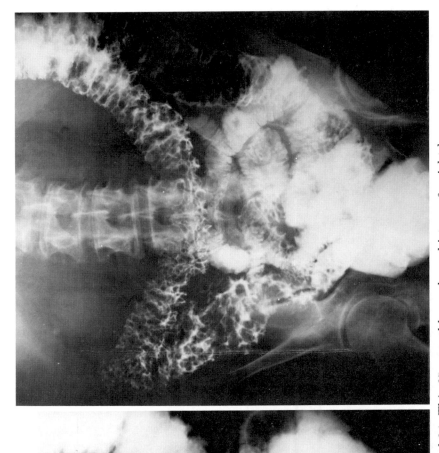
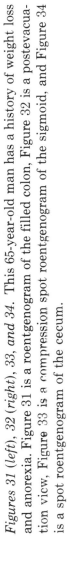

Figures 31 (left), 32 (right), 33, and 34. This 65-year-old man has a history of weight loss and anorexia. Figure 31 is a roentgenogram of the filled colon, Figure 32 is a postevacuation view, Figure 33 is a compression spot roentgenogram of the sigmoid, and Figure 34 is a spot roentgenogram of the cecum.

Questions 69 through 72

69. Which one of the following is the *MOST* likely diagnosis?

   (A) Familial polyposis
   (B) Granulomatous colitis
   (C) Ulcerative colitis
   (D) Lymphosarcoma
   (E) Colitis cystica profunda

70. Which one of the following is *LEAST* characteristic of familial polyposis?

   (A) Involvement of the small bowel
   (B) Development of carcinoma before age 40
   (C) Tiny sessile polypoid lesions
   (D) Absence of rigidity
   (E) Normal length and caliber of the colon

71. Which one of the following roentgenographic findings is *LEAST* common in granulomatous colitis?

   (A) Involvement of the rectum
   (B) Associated involvement of the terminal ileum
   (C) Large pseudopolyps
   (D) Limitation to the right half of the colon
   (E) "Skip" areas

72. Which one of the following is the *MOST* common manifestation of lymphoma of the colon?

   (A) Multiple small polypoid lesions
   (B) Single large bulky mass
   (C) Diffuse infiltration of the wall
   (D) Multiple ulcerations
   (E) Obstruction

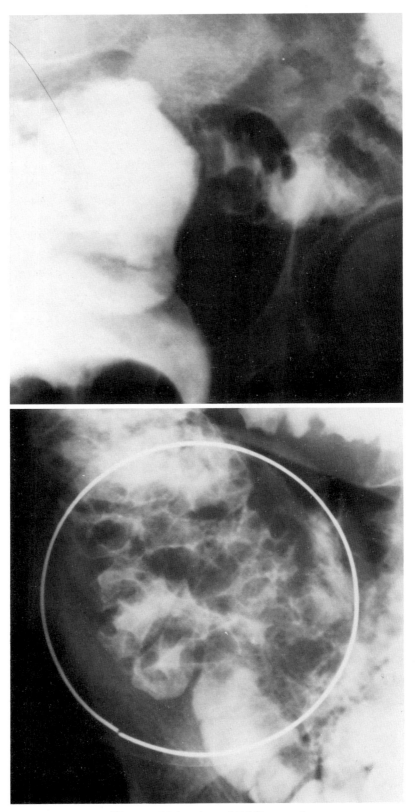

Figures 33 (top) and 34 (bottom)

Discussion

QUESTION 69

The correct diagnosis is lymphosarcoma (D). The roentgenograms show multiple scattered small (2 to 10 mm.) polypoid lesions along the superior and inferior aspects of the transverse colon (Figure 34A, "A" *arrows*), as well as a few such small polypoid protuberances seen face on (Figure 34A, "B" *arrows*). Some of these can also be seen on the postevacuation film (Figure 34B, *arrows*). In the cecal and sigmoid areas the same type of lesion is seen (Figures 33 and 34) but the nodules appear larger and almost suggest multiple prominent mucosal folds. Multiple small nodular lesions of this kind are one of the typical, even though infrequent, manifestations of lymphoma of the colon. The relative uniformity of shape of the lesions throughout the colon, their relatively equal size, and the patient's age are in favor of the diagnosis of lymphosarcoma as contrasted with familial polyposis which in this case would be the most difficult roentgenological differential diagnosis.

The incidence of malignancy of the colon in familial multiple polyposis is so high that most patients, if untreated, do not survive beyond the age of 50 years. Granulomatous colitis and ulcerative colitis are both excluded by absence of involvement of the wall of the colon itself: polypoid protuberances may develop in both of these diseases as a result of the combination of extensive ulceration and hyperplastic edematous changes in the remaining mucosa—they are like islands of hyperplastic inflamed mucosa in a sea of ulceration. However, in both these diseases, there are changes in the shape of the colon, particularly involving loss of haustrations either in the entire colon or parts of it, as well as shortening and rigidity. In contrast, with the polypoid type of lymphoma as seen in this case, and with familial polyposis, the overall shape of the colon remains normal. Colitis cystica profunda is a lesion which primarily affects the rectum. It is also not a true polyposis but rather results in a lumpy polypoid appearance of the mucosa as a result of a cystic inflammatory process in the wall of this part of the colon.

QUESTION 70

Small bowel involvement is least characteristic of familial polyposis and the correct answer is, therefore, (A). Familial polyposis is an inheritable disease, transmitted according to a simple mendelian dominant. The lesions occur entirely or almost entirely in the colon. They are most

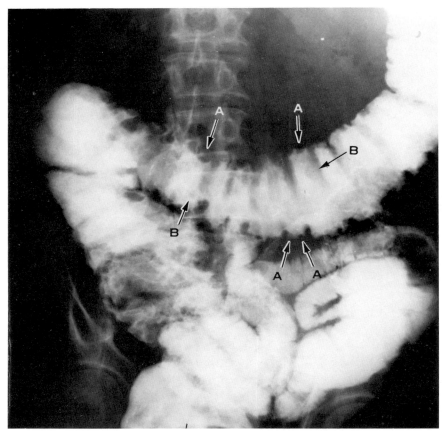

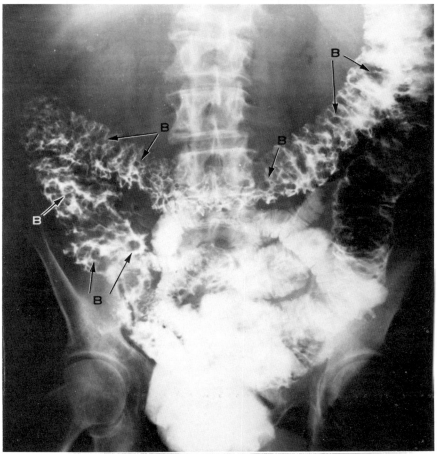

Figure 34A (top) and B (bottom)

prominently present in the rectum and sigmoid. Hence the diagnosis can generally be made through sigmoidoscopy. In many cases, the colon is filled with a myriad of very small polyps. In others, there is some variation and the largest polyps in this disease may be up to several centimeters in diameter. Thus, tiny sessile polypoid lesions (C) is in many cases a true description of the disease. The incidence of malignant degeneration is very high and is felt to occur roughly some 20 years earlier than the average carcinoma of the large bowel (B). Characteristically, the colon is quite flexible and is normal except for the presence of the multiple polyps and, when the time arrives, the presence of carcinoma. Hence, (D) is a true statement but not a correct answer to this question. (E) refers again to the normal overall appearances of the colon in this disease except for the presence of the polypoid lesions. The reader is referred to the review by Calabro for a discussion of the more common familial polyposis syndromes.

QUESTION 71

The correct answer is involvement of the rectum (A). As one reads the appropriate literature in the last few years, the diagnostic borderline between ulcerative and granulomatous colitis is becoming a bit indistinct. Nevertheless, of the offered choices, involvement of the rectum occurs least commonly in granulomatous colitis. The ileum is commonly involved (B) since the disease frequently is an enterocolitis rather than a pure colitis. Pseudopolyps (C) of various sizes can develop both in ulcerative and in granulomatous colitis. The right colon is predominantly involved in granulomatous colitis. Limitation to the right half of the colon (D) is fairly common and skip areas (E) occur characteristically both in regional enteritis and in granulomatous colitis.

QUESTION 72

A single, sometimes large and occasionally multilobulated mass is the most common manifestation of lymphoma in the colon (B). The multiple small polypoid lesions (A), as in this case, the diffuse infiltration of the wall (C), and multiple ulcerations (D) are all found in colon lymphoma, and sometimes suggest the diagnosis of lymphoma rather than carcinoma. But as far as overall numbers are concerned, the single mass is predominant in frequency. This in fact makes it essentially impossible to separate roentgenologically most lymphomas of the colon from carcinomas preoperatively unless associated findings in other organs are present. The same to some extent is true of the multiple small polypoid lesions seen in this case—the exact diagnosis is often not known until the lesions are biopsied or surgical exploration is performed.

The frequency of lymphomatous involvement of the gastrointestinal tract generally decreases in descending order from the more proximal to the more distal portions. Lymphomas of the colon are infrequent. In view of the frequency of carcinomatous and adenomatous processes in this organ it is difficult to establish the diagnosis of lymphoma on a roentgenographic basis alone. The most common manifestation is the single large bulky mass, followed in frequency by diffuse infiltration of the wall, multiple small polypoid lesions, and, lastly, especially in youngsters, paradoxical dilatation of the organ.

The lesions are generally relatively soft and flexible. Therefore, obstruction is distinctly less common with lymphoma than with carcinoma. Intussusception may occasionally lead to acute clinical problems with obstruction. The cecum is involved most often; the rectum, sigmoid, and transverse colon follow in that order.

The differential diagnosis of multiple small polypoid lesions is also quite difficult on a roentgenological basis alone. The inflammatory lesions (ulcerative and granulomatous colitis) can be separated out by virtue of their involvement of the wall and loss of haustral pattern of the colon, as well as shortening and abnormal shape.

An important differential diagnosis is lymphoid hyperplasia in children which is an entirely benign condition. In this entity the nodules are rather small, sessile, and sometimes umbilicated.

One also needs to be aware of the occurrence of benign lymphoid hyperplasia in the lower ileum which occurs in some patients with familial polyposis and with Gardner's syndrome as well. This is important because it may save the patient unnecessary resection of portions of the lower small bowel for what turns out to be a purely benign lesion and *is not part* of the polyposis process itself.

SUGGESTED READINGS

LYMPHOMA OF THE COLON
1. Wolf BS, Marshak RH: Roentgen features of diffuse lymphosarcoma of colon. Radiology 75:733–740, 1960
2. Wychulis AR, Beahrs OH, Woolner LB: Malignant lymphoma of the colon. A study of 69 cases. Arch Surg 93:215–225, 1966

MULTIPLE POLYPOID LESIONS AND DIFFERENTIAL DIAGNOSIS
1. Calabro JJ: Hereditable multiple polyposis syndromes of the gastrointestinal tract. Am J Med 33:276–281, 1962
2. Cronkhite LW Jr, Canada WJ: Generalized gastrointestinal polyposis. New England J Med 252:1014–1015, 1955

3. Franken EA Jr: Lymphoid hyperplasia of the colon. Radiology *94:*329–334, 1970
4. Koehler PR, Kyaw MM, Fenlon JW: Diffuse gastrointestinal polyposis and ectodermal changes. Radiology *103:*589–594, 1972
5. Marshak RH, Moseley JE, Wolf BS: Roentgen findings in familial polyposis with special emphasis on differential diagnosis. Radiology *80:*374–382, 1963
6. Ross P: Gardner's syndrome. Am J Roentgenol *96:*298–301, 1966
7. Schaupp WC, Volpe PA: Management of diffuse colonic polyposis. Am J Surg *124:*218–222, 1972
8. Vanhoutte JJ: Polypoid lymphoid hyperplasia of terminal ileum in patients with familial polyposis coli and with Gardner's syndrome. Am J Roentgenol *110:*340–342, 1970

COLITIS CYSTICA PROFUNDA
See bibliography on p. 52

CORRECT ANSWERS

Question 69-(D)
Question 70-(A)
Question 71-(A)
Question 72-(B)

NOTES

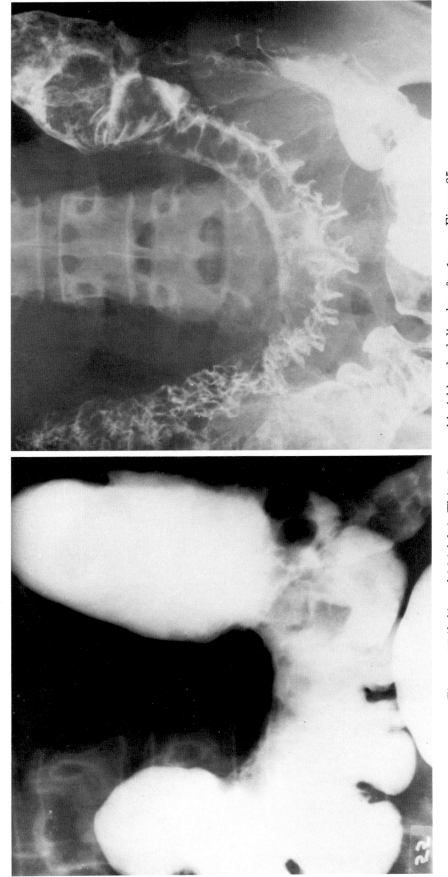

Figures 35 (left) and 36 (right). This 15-year-old girl has had diarrhea for 1 year. Figure 35 is a roentgenogram of the filled transverse colon, and Figure 36 is a postevacuation view.

Questions 73 through 77

73. Which one of the following is the *MOST* likely diagnosis?

   (A) Ulcerative colitis
   (B) Granulomatous colitis
   (C) Polyposis
   (D) Peutz-Jeghers syndrome
   (E) Scleroderma

74. Which one of the following is *MOST* suggestive of ulcerative colitis?

   (A) Pseudodiverticula
   (B) Eccentric involvement
   (C) Undermining ulcers
   (D) Stenotic disease of the terminal ileum
   (E) Predominant involvement of the right side of the colon

75. In the differential diagnosis of ulcerative and granulomatous colitis, which one of the following statements is *LEAST* likely?

   (A) Toxic megacolon is diagnostic of ulcerative colitis
   (B) Granulomatous colitis generally occurs in a younger age group than ulcerative colitis
   (C) Carcinoma of the colon is a more common complication of ulcerative than of granulomatous colitis
   (D) Distal colonic involvement is less characteristic of granulomatous than of ulcerative colitis
   (E) Massive hemorrhage may occur in both ulcerative and granulomatous colitis

76. Which one of the following is *MOST* characteristic of familial polyposis?

   (A) It is first discovered in infancy
   (B) The polyps are usually greater than 1 cm. in diameter
   (C) Carcinoma frequently develops before middle age
   (D) Hemorrhage occurs frequently
   (E) There are associated small bowel polyps

77. Which one of the following statements concerning Peutz-Jeghers syndrome is *LEAST* likely?

   (A) The polyps may be seen in the stomach
   (B) The polyps are hamartomas and not adenomas
   (C) Malignancy is unusual
   (D) The polyps only occur in the small intestine
   (E) Skin lesions are associated

Discussion

QUESTION 73

   The correct answer to question 73 is (B) since these illustrations show some characteristic roentgen findings of granulomatous colitis. Note the long area of involvement (*arrows*, Figure 36A) on the superior aspect of the transverse colon which has an indistinct curvilinear margin in striking contrast to the sharply outlined large sac-like haustra ("*H*" in Figure 36A) seen on the opposite inferior aspect. The rigid-appearing curvilinear superior aspect of the transverse colon and the irregular contour indicate destruction of the normal mucosa. This relatively long diseased segment and the eccentric involvement of the superior aspect of the transverse colon are highly suggestive of an inflammatory process. There is also a similar, not so easily recognized area of involvement in the descending colon (*white arrows*, Figure 36B). Between these two areas of involvement, the splenic flexure region is seen to be of normal caliber and contour. Some fecal material is present, particularly in the splenic flexure area (vigorous preparation of the colon was not carried out because of the patient's diarrhea). The eccentric nature of the disease can be appreciated by comparing the behavior of the large sac-like filled haustra ("*H*" in Figure 36A) on the inferior aspect of the transverse colon, which contract normally ("*H*" in Figure 36B), as compared to the unchanging curvilinear configuration of the involved rigid superior aspect of the transverse colon (*arrows* in Figures 36A and B). Of great interest on the postevacuation view is the linear barium collection (*vertical black arrows*, Figure 36B) which is a large, tangentially seen, *longitudinally oriented* fissure-like ulcer in the rigid thickened superior aspect of the transverse colon. The large amount of barium in the lumen on the filled view obscures this marginal barium collection. The gross specimen of this case clearly shows a longitudinally oriented deep ulcer (*between long black vertical arrows, right side* of Figure 36C). There are also two longitudinal ulcers on the left side of the specimen (*upper and lower rows of vertical arrows, left side* of Figure 36C). Such ulcers are actually in the form of deep fissures in the markedly thickened wall of the colon.

Now, please refer to the postevacuation roentgenogram again and note the several transversely oriented linear streaks of barium (*small black arrows*, Figure 36B) which are fissure-like *transverse* ulcers so characteristic of granulomatous colitis. Several of these transverse ulcers (*horizontal black arrows*, Figure 36C) are particularly apparent as they traverse the area *between* the two longitudinal ulcers indicated by the *vertical arrows on the left side* of the gross specimen. There are also wider transverse ulcers (*horizontal arrows*) extending *downward* from the large longitudinal ulcer on the right side of the gross specimen. Note that all of the visible mucosa, even that *immediately adjacent* to the deep longitudinal and transverse ulcers, although somewhat edematous and "polypoid" in appearance, is of virtually *normal* color, in contrast to the often intense injection seen in ulcerative colitis (see *black areas* in Figures 2D and E, pp. 9 and 10). The markedly *thickened* wall of the colon in granulomatous colitis makes possible the development of such *deep* fissure-like ulcers. Thus, the two roentgenograms in this case clearly show some important radiological features of granulomatous colitis; i.e., "skip" areas of disease, the eccentric type of involvement, and the longitudinal and transverse ulcers.

Ulcerative colitis would be an unlikely diagnosis in this case because of the presence of *two* areas of disease separated by the normal-appearing splenic flexure, in contrast to the characteristic *continuous* involvement of only *one* diseased segment in ulcerative colitis (see Figures 1 and 2, pp. 2 and 4). Although in some cases of granulomatous colitis the entire circumference may be involved, the eccentric nature of the changes shown here is also in contrast to the circumferential nature of the involvement which is so characteristic of ulcerative colitis (see Figures 1 and 2, pp. 2 and 4). Although the "collar-button" (Figure 2C, p. 8) or spicule-shaped ulcers (*arrows*, Fig. 2A, p. 6) are frequently seen in ulcerative colitis, they *sometimes* occur in granulomatous colitis, too. However, the deep longitudinal and transverse fissure-like ulcers shown here are virtually diagnostic of granulomatous colitis.

Although the areas of mucosa demarcated by the surrounding *intercon-*

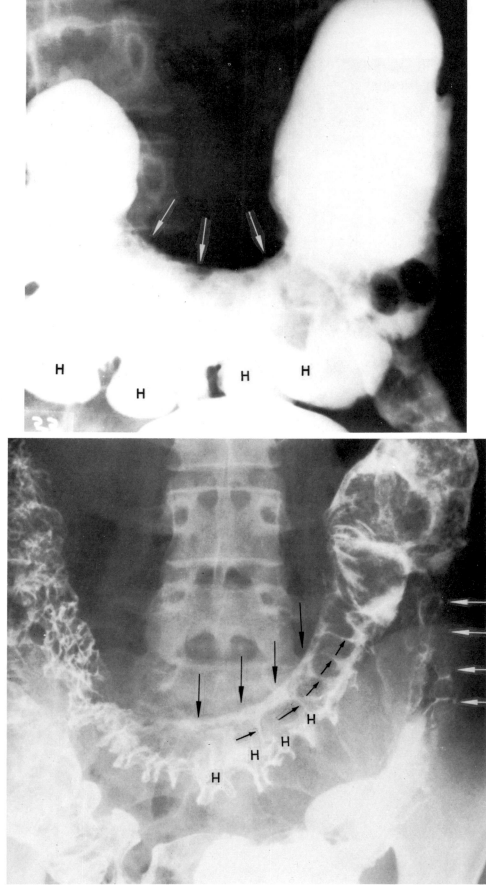

Figure 36A (top) and B (bottom)

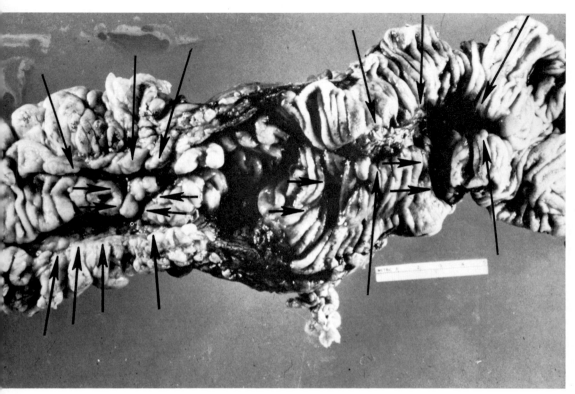

Figure 36C

nected longitudinal and transverse ulcers simulate rather large polyps (Figure 36), they are somewhat rectangular in shape, fairly similar in size, and oriented in a single row. Thus, they do not look like true adenomatous polyps which are rounder, variable in size, and not oriented in rows. Of course, the characteristic longitudinal and transverse ulcers would also militate against the diagnosis of adenomatous polyps. Adenomatous polyps which occur in the colon are generally few in number and scattered, rather than being localized to one area and are not lined up in a row like the "pseudopolyps" or "cobblestones" shown in the transverse colon in this case. Furthermore, the obvious *rigidity* of most of the superior wall of the transverse colon would not be a feature of polyposis of any kind.

The Peutz-Jeghers syndrome is usually manifested by hamartomatous and/or adenomatous polyps in the stomach and small intestine, but they do not ordinarily occur in the colon.

Scleroderma may involve the colon in far advanced cases and the loss of smooth muscle in this disease may result in enough weakening of the affected wall of the colon to permit the formation of unusual square-shaped "pseudodiverticula" which are thought to be characteristic of scleroderma. In the case shown here the prominent haustral pattern on the inferior aspect of the transverse colon certainly resembles the wide-necked, sac-like type of "pseudodiverticula" which have been described in the small intestine and colon of patients who have scleroderma. However, in this case of granulomatous colitis, the large sac-like haustra are probably due to exaggerated deep contractions of the intact circular muscle of the uninvolved inferior aspect of the transverse colon in response to the *stimulus* of the inflammatory disease involving the extensive parts of the *opposite* superior aspect of the transverse colon. Furthermore, these barium-filled diverticula-like haustra ("*H*" in Figure 36A) contract normally ("*H*" in Figure 36B) on the postevacuation view, in rather striking contrast to the *absence* of contractions which is so characteristic of the "pseudodiverticula" seen in scleroderma owing to the replacement of muscle tissue by fibrous tissue. Thus, the "pseudodiverticula" which occur in scleroderma are often *best* seen on postevacuation views, since the failure of the haustra to contract causes them to remain filled with barium, in contrast to other areas of the colon which contract and empty normally. Furthermore, longitudinal or transverse ulcerations are not seen in scleroderma, and eccentric rigidity of the bowel wall is not a feature of this disease.

QUESTION 74

The correct answer to question 74 is (C). Of all the responses listed the one which is *most* suggestive of ulcerative colitis is undermined ulcers. The other listed responses refer to *characteristic* features of granulomatous colitis. Although undermined ulcers may occasionally be seen in granulomatous colitis, this is the only one of the listed responses which can *also* occur in ulcerative colitis. "Pseudodiverticula" are seen in scleroderma and granulomatous colitis, but are not associated with ulcerative colitis. Furthermore, eccentric involvement is not characteristic of ulcerative colitis, whereas it is quite characteristic of granulomatous disease as illustrated in this case. Stenotic disease of the terminal ileum is not seen in ulcerative colitis, but the opposite type of involvement is seen; i.e., a "backwash" ileitis which consists of a patulous, often slightly *dilated* terminal ileum (see "*T.I.*" in Figure 2B, p. 7) with a wide patent ileocecal valve. Predominant right-sided colon involvement is also not typical for ulcerative colitis, and although such right-sided localization may occur in a few cases, involvement of the left side of the colon is much more characteristic of this disease. Since both ulcerative colitis and granulomatous colitis can occasionally involve the *entire* colon, the appearance of the terminal ileum can be of *decisive* importance in making the correct differential diagnosis between these two conditions.

QUESTION 75

The correct answer to question 75 is (A). Of the various statements concerning the differential diagnosis between ulcerative and granulomatous colitis, the *least* likely one is that which states that toxic megacolon is *diagnostic* of ulcerative colitis. Toxic megacolon is, indeed, a common and dreaded complication of ulcerative colitis, but it is *not* diagnostic of that disease. It is also seen in patients with necrotizing enterocolitis, and it may occur as a serious complication following the administration of parasympathomimetic drugs. When toxic megacolon *does* occur in ulcerative colitis, it is believed by many radiologists that a barium enema is contraindicated because of the added danger of perforation; i.e., since the danger of *spontaneous* perforation is *already* great owing to the distended, thin friable wall of the colon, any increase in intraluminal pressure which may occur during a barium enema may be the "straw that breaks the camel's back", so to speak, with resulting perforation. Since all of the other statements in question 75 are *true*, they are, therefore, *wrong* answers.

QUESTION 76

The correct answer to question 76 is (C). Of the responses listed in this question the one which is *most* characteristic of familial polyposis is that which states that carcinoma frequently develops before middle age. The other statements about familial polyposis are *false*, and, therefore, *incorrect*. Most cases of familial polyposis are discovered during the *late teens or early adulthood*, rather than being first discovered during infancy. Furthermore, the polyps are characteristically less than 1 cm. in diameter, often being so tiny and numerous that the overall appearance of the profiled margin of the colon is rather "fuzzy" or "velvety". Although *small* amounts of blood may occasionally be seen in the stools, gross hemorrhages are rare. Familial polyposis is *not* associated with small bowel polyps, although in some cases there may be an associated lymphoid hyperplasia in the terminal ileum, the hyperplastic lymphoid follicles having the appearance of tiny "polyps". The explanation for the lymphoid hyperplasia occasionally associated with familial polyposis is unknown, but possibly it is related to the fact that this disease may be of a viral etiology. Thus, the presence of such a generalized viral inflammatory disease of the colon could explain the lymphoid hyperplasia in the contiguous terminal ileum.

QUESTION 77

The correct answer to question 77 is (D). Although polyps are *often* seen in the small intestine in the Peutz-Jeghers syndrome, the polyps are *not* limited to that part of the gastrointestinal tract. They are *often* seen in the stomach, but are *rarely* seen in the colon. The polyps in this condition are almost always hamartomatous in nature and malignancy is unusual. Pigmented areas at the mucocutaneous junctions of the lips and anus are an important feature of the Peutz-Jeghers syndrome.

DISCUSSION

It should be remembered that the differentiation between granulomatous disease (Crohn's disease) of the colon and ulcerative colitis depends upon the careful evaluation of *all* available clinical, radiological, and pathological information. The final distinction between these two diseases will rarely rest on any *one* roentgenological, sigmoidoscopic, clinical, or pathological finding since there is a certain amount of overlap of all findings which are *claimed* to be "characteristic" by *each* discipline (see Table 1, p. 14, for the tabulation of the differential diagnostic criteria of these two diseases). Thus, some cases of granulomatous colitis may be roentgenologically indistinguishable from ulcerative colitis, particularly when the entire colon is involved. Furthermore, a small number of cases of ulcerative colitis involve predominantly the *right side* of the colon and, thus, may simulate granulomatous disease. The ulcers may also be somewhat similar in appearance in both diseases, although the classical undermining which produces the "collar-button" type of ulcers is probably *more commonly* associated with ulcerative colitis. Conversely, clear-cut longitudinal and transverse linear ulcers are virtually never seen in patients with ulcerative colitis, but are common in granulomatous colitis. Similarly, although in the *majority* of cases the clinical features may be in favor of one or the other of these diseases, the use of clinical methods alone will result in failure to make the correct diagnosis in a certain number of cases. Examination of *pathologic* tissue will also fail to establish the correct diagnosis in some cases because "typical" granulomatous changes may occasionally be seen in ulcerative colitis, whereas such "characteristic" findings may be missing in some cases of granulomatous colitis!

SUGGESTED READINGS

GRANULOMATOUS COLITIS *VERSUS* ULCERATIVE COLITIS
See bibliography on page 16

POLYPOSIS
1. Dukes CE, Lockhart-Mummery HE: Familial intestinal polyposis. Surg Clin North Am 35:1277–1281, 1965

2. Marshak RH, Moseley JE, Wolf BS: The roentgen findings in familial polyposis with special emphasis on differential diagnosis. Radiology *80:*374–382, 1963
3. Smith WG: Multiple polyposis, Gardner's syndrome and desmoid tumors. Dis Colon & Rectum *1:*323–332, 1958
4. Weiner RS, Cooper P: Multiple polyposis of the colon, osteomatosis and soft-tissue tumors. Report of a familial syndrome. New England J Med *253:*795–799, 1955

PEUTZ-JEGHERS SYNDROME

1. Farmer RG, Hawk WA, Turnbull RB: The spectrum of the Peutz-Jeghers syndrome. Report of 3 cases. Am J Digestive Dis NS *8:*953–961, 1963
2. Horn RC, Payne WA, Fine G: The Peutz-Jeghers syndrome (gastrointestinal polyposis with mucocutaneous pigmentation). Report of a case terminating with disseminated gastrointestinal cancer. Arch Pathol *76:*29–37, 1963

SCLERODERMA

1. Hale CH, Schatzki R: Roentgenological appearance of the gastrointestinal tract in scleroderma. Am J Roentgenol *51:*407–420, 1944
2. Meszaros WT: The colon in systemic sclerosis (scleroderma). Am J Roentgenol *82:*1000–1002, 1959
3. Queloz JM, Woloshin HJ: Sacculation of the small intestine in scleroderma. Radiology *105:*513–515, 1972

CORRECT ANSWERS

Question 73-(B)
Question 74-(C)
Question 75-(A)
Question 76-(C)
Question 77-(D)

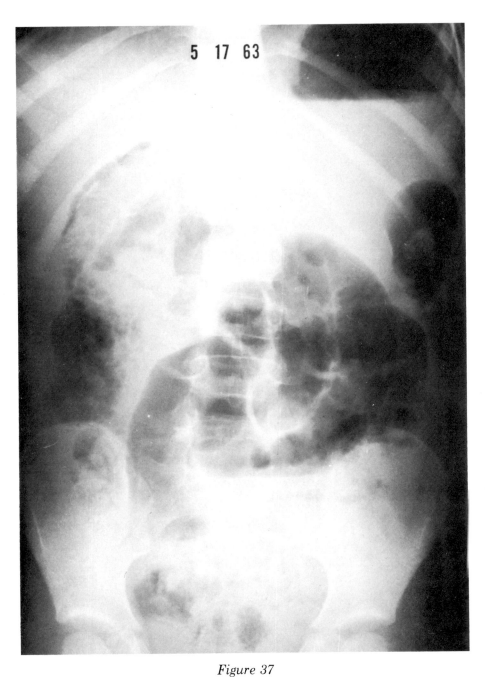

Figure 37

Figures 37 and 38. This 10-year-old boy has complained of abdominal pain for 2 days. Roentgenograms of the abdomen were taken with the patient in the upright (Figure 37) and supine (Figure 38) positions.

Questions 78 and 79

78. Which one of the following is the *MOST* likely diagnosis?

    (A) Pneumatosis coli
    (B) Small bowel obstruction
    (C) Retroperitoneal hematoma
    (D) Retroperitoneal perforation of the duodenum
    (E) Intramural hematoma of the colon

79. Which one of the following roentgenographic findings is *LEAST* significant in the diagnosis of retroperitoneal hematoma?

    (A) Obliteration of psoas muscle shadow
    (B) Presence of a soft tissue mass
    (C) Lateral displacement of the kidney
    (D) Displacement of the duodenum
    (E) Fractures of lumbar transverse processes

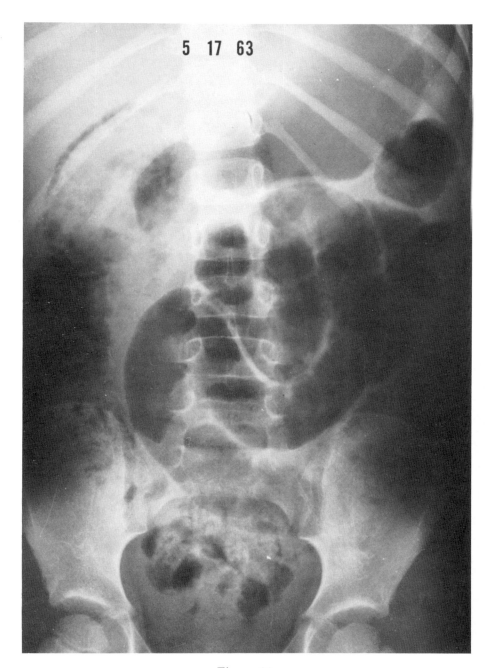

Figure 38

Discussion

Figures 37 and 38 demonstrate abnormal gas bubbles within the right upper quadrant, dilated small bowel loops, and a dilated air- and fluid-filled stomach. In addition, there appears to be gas outlining the lateral border of the right kidney. The gas bubbles stay fixed in both the upright (Figure 37) and recumbent (Figure 38) films which suggests that they do not lie within bowel but almost assuredly within the retroperitoneal space. Of the possible answers listed in question 78, **retroperitoneal perforation of the duodenum (D) is the most likely diagnosis.** Although the dilated stomach and duodenum should make ruptured duodenum your primary diagnosis, other causes of retroperitoneal abscess cannot be excluded from the plain films alone.

A bit of clinical information was withheld, i.e., a history of trauma. Although a history of trauma can usually be obtained in cases of bowel injury, in many reported cases the injury was so mild as to have been overlooked or forgotten. It is, therefore, the radiologist who often suggests the diagnosis, and early diagnosis is vital since the mortality is 75 to 90 per cent in improperly diagnosed and treated cases of duodenal rupture.

Traumatic rupture and hematoma of the duodenum are more prevalent in children than in adults; and as would be expected, boys are more commonly affected than girls. The second portion of the duodenum, the jejunum at the ligament of Treitz, the terminal ileum, cecum, and rectosigmoid areas are relatively fixed and, therefore, are most susceptible to injury.

The one possible differential diagnosis listed in question 78 which may have given some difficulty is pneumatosis coli (Figure 38A). The grape-like bubbles outlining the wall of the colon seem similar in appearance to those demonstrated in Figures 37 and 38. However, this is a benign condition and as such is most often found incidentally and not because of significant complaints of pain. Barium enema will confirm the diagnosis of pneumatosis coli (Figure 38B and Figure 7, p. 42). More detailed description of this condition is present on p. 48–51.

Duodenal rupture is almost invariably associated with hematoma of the duodenum. Administering a water soluble contrast medium may not demonstrate the site of perforation but will usually reveal the hematoma. The roentgen picture is one of deformity of the duodenum (*large arrows*, Figures

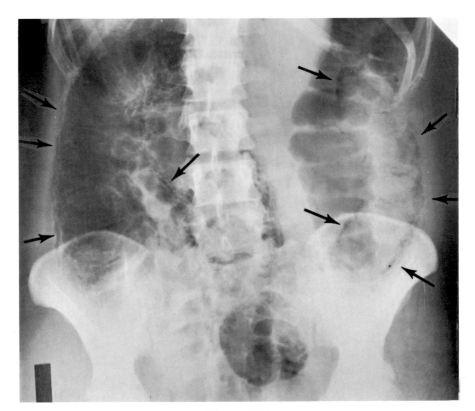

Figure 38A

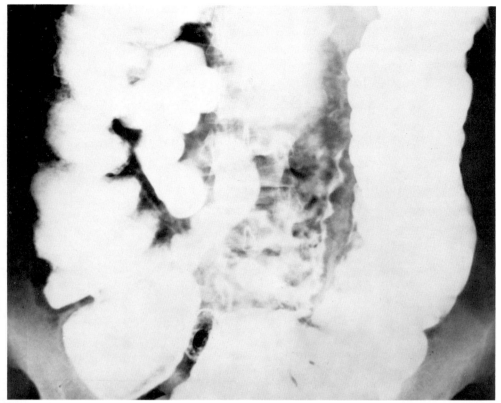

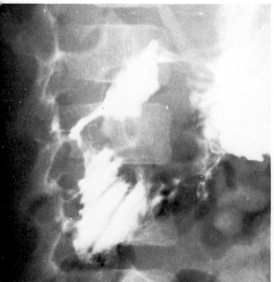

Figure 38C

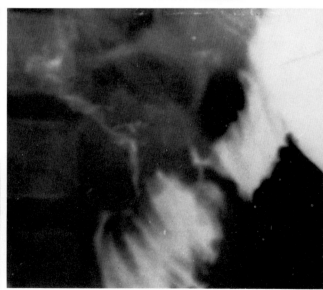

Figure 38D

Questions 78 and 79 / 189

38C and D). Sometimes there may be evidence of an intramural mass, although in the case presented here there was a somewhat annular narrowing in the mid portion of the duodenum (Figure 38C) probably due to a combination of intramural and extramural bleeding. The associated large folds proximal and distal to this annular deformity (lower right quadrant of the lateral view, Figure 38D) are no doubt due to submucosal hemorrhage (see discussion of "transverse ridging" on p. 140, and Figure 28A, *left arrows*). The actual site of the perforation is well demonstrated by an irregular fistulous tract (which is seen extending upward and posteriorly into the left upper quadrant of the lateral view, Figure 38D). The appearance of gas around the right kidney following blunt abdominal trauma is so characteristic that the diagnosis should be immediately suggested on the basis of the plain abdominal radiographs alone.

QUESTION 79

All of the possibilities listed in question 79 may be seen with retroperitoneal hematoma. Because **absence of a psoas shadow (A)** in a perfectly well patient is not uncommon this sign would be least contributory in arriving at a correct diagnosis. In a study by Elkin and Cohen, 22 per cent of normal patients had a poorly visualized right psoas and 9 per cent had nonvisualization. On the left side, the figures were 15 and 5 per cent respectively.

SUGGESTED READINGS

1. Elkin M, Cohen G: Diagnostic value of the psoas shadow. J Faculty Radiol *13–14*:210–217, 1962–1963
2. Felson B, Levin EJ: Intramural hematoma of the duodenum. Radiology *63*:823–831, 1954
3. Gould J, Thorwarth WT: Retroperitoneal rupture of the duodenum due to blurt non-penetrating abdominal trauma. Radiology *80*:743–747, 1963
4. McCort JJ: Radiologic examination in blunt abdominal trauma. Radiol Clin North Am *2*:121–143, 1964
5. Nelson JF: The roentgenologic evaluation of abdominal trauma. Radiol Clin North Am *4*:415–431, 1966
6. Wiot JF: Intramural small intestinal hemorrhage—differential diagnosis. Semin in Roentgenol *1*:219–233, 1966

CORRECT ANSWERS

Question 78-(D)
Question 79-(A)

NOTES

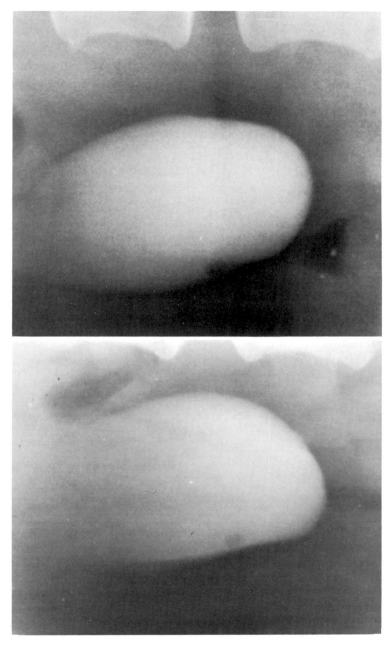

Figures 39 (left) and 40 (right). This 60-year-old woman has had vague epigastric distress for several years. Roentgenograms of the gallbladder were taken with the patient in the prone (Figure 39) and upright (Figure 40) positions.

Questions 80 through 85

80. Which one of the following is the *MOST* likely diagnosis?

    (A) Adenomyoma
    (B) Gallstone
    (C) Cholesterol polyp
    (D) Adenomatous polyp
    (E) Carcinoma

81. Which one of the following statements is *INCORRECT*?

    (A) Unconjugated Telepaque is fat soluble
    (B) Orally-administered Telepaque is absorbed by the intestinal mucosa
    (C) After absorption, Telepaque is bound to serum albumin
    (D) The Telepaque excreted into the bile is water soluble
    (E) Conjugated Telepaque is easily absorbed by the intestinal mucosa

82. Which one of the following procedures is the single *MOST* helpful part of intravenous cholangiography?

    (A) Roentgenography of the erect patient
    (B) Right lateral decubitus roentgenography
    (C) Tomography
    (D) Compression roentgenography
    (E) Roentgenography after a fatty meal

83. In a patient who has *not* had a cholecystectomy, which one of the following disorders is indicated by good visualization of the common bile duct without corresponding visualization of the gallbladder during cholangiography?

    (A) Carcinoma of the ampulla of Vater
    (B) Stone impacted in the distal common bile duct
    (C) Obstruction of the cystic duct
    (D) Carcinoma of the pancreas
    (E) None of the above

84. Which one of the following statements concerning cholesterol polyps is *MOST* likely?

(A) They are precancerous
(B) They usually are large
(C) They are easily distinguished from papillomas
(D) They commonly occur in or near the cystic duct
(E) They commonly are multiple

85. Which one of the following conditions is *LEAST* likely to be associated with an increased incidence of gallstones?

(A) Hypercholesterolemia
(B) Sickle cell anemia
(C) Diabetes mellitus
(D) Chronic cholecystitis
(E) Gout

Discussion

QUESTION 80

Figures 39 and 40 demonstrate a fixed filling defect along the lateral wall of a normally visualized gallbladder representing a **cholesterol polyp (C)**. The differential diagnosis of such a lesion is extensive and must include cholesterol polyp, inflammatory polyp, mucosal adenoma, adenomyoma, fixed stone, polypoid malignant tumor, and a few other rare entities. On a statistical basis alone, however, cholesterol polyp is the most common fixed lesion in this area.

The term adenomyoma is a misnomer as it is not a true neoplasm but rather a localized form of adenomyomatosis. Adenomyomatosis is also called cholecystitis glandularis proliferans and represents hyperplasia of the gallbladder wall, the result of proliferation of surface epithelium and thickening of the muscle layer. Adenomyoma almost invariably presents within the fundus of the gallbladder. It is characterized cholecystographically by a filling defect representing the mass projecting from the wall into the lumen, an opaque central speck of contrast medium representing umbilication of the mound, and opaque dots representing diverticula at the

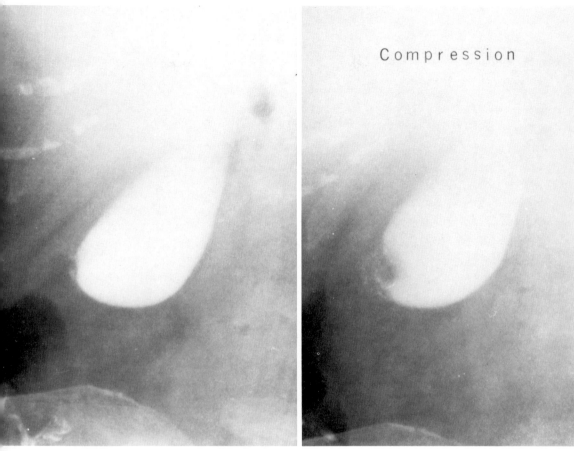

Compression

Figure 40A   Figure 40B

periphery of the nodule. Overdistention of the gallbladder may result in failure to demonstrate the mass but shows only the central area of umbilication (Figure 40A). With compression, the mass of the adenomyoma may be visualized as well as the surrounding contrast-filled diverticula (Figure 40B).

Although on a single recumbent film the defect could well have represented a gallstone, its failure to descend on the upright film and the absence of other stones make this a poor diagnostic choice. An adenomatous polyp would certainly have to be given consideration as it *cannot* be differentiated radiographically from a cholesterol polyp, but again the much greater incidence of cholesterol polyp makes this the more likely diagnosis.

Carcinoma of the gallbladder is almost invariably associated with chronic gallbladder disease and stones, and cholecystographic demonstration of the neoplasm is rare. It is interesting that in a 15-year follow-up of 226 cases of polypoid lesions of the gallbladder (as reported by Ochsner), there were no deaths from gallbladder carcinoma nor was carcinoma *in situ* demonstrated.

QUESTION 81

Unconjugated Telepaque and other cholecystographic media are readily absorbed by the intestinal mucosa; whereas the injectable media, such as Cholografin, are poorly absorbed. This difference in absorption ability is related to the fact that Telepaque is lipid soluble whereas Cholografin and other injectable solutions are soluble in aqueous solutions only. For this reason, once Telepaque is absorbed and bound to the serum albumin and conjugated within the liver to form the glucuronide ester it becomes water soluble. As such it is poorly absorbed by intestinal mucosa except in unusual circumstances. **Thus, your answer to question 81 should be (E).**

QUESTION 82

Although all of the answers in question 82 are correct in that they are helpful in certain situations, tomography appears to be the *most* beneficial adjunct to routine filming during intravenous cholangiography. **Your answer to question 82,** therefore, **should be (C).**

In many patients, visualization of the biliary system on conventional radiographs is so poor that only tomography can provide disclosure of a stone or dilation of the duct. In addition, it is recommended that even in the case of nonvisualization of the duct or gallbladder with conventional films that tomography be performed.

QUESTION 83

Good visualization of a normal common bile duct and nonvisualization of the gallbladder with intravenous cholangiography are almost invariably an indication of **cystic duct obstruction (C).** If common duct obstruction and dilation exist for any cause, the gallbladder may not visualize even if the cystic duct is not obstructed. When this occurs, common duct visualization is predictably poor and frequently there is also cystic duct obstruction. The use of intravenous cholangiography in an attempt to differentiate acute pancreatitis from acute cholecystitis is based on this finding, since the latter is almost invariably associated with cystic duct obstruction.

QUESTION 84

The cholesterol polyp is a greatly enlarged villous-like structure covered with a single layer of epithelium and contains no glandular elements. It is filled largely with macrophages ladened with cholesterol esters. Many are attached with delicate stalks and the ease with which they can be detached has led some to postulate that they may be precursors to gallstones. Generally they are quite small as seen in this case and they are frequently multiple. The cholesterol polyp has no predilection for any portion of the gallbladder and has no malignant potential. **Your answer,** therefore, **to question 84 should be (E).**

QUESTION 85

In question 85 patients with all of the listed conditions except **gout (E)** have a greater incidence of gallstones than the general population. Hypercholesterolemia is a well-known cause as is sickle cell anemia because of the hemolytic aspect of the latter disease. The incidence of gallstones in a postmortem series of diabetics is about 25 per cent, whereas in the general population it is about 8 per cent. Chronic cholecystitis is, of course, a frequent concomitant of gallstones. Other conditions apparently associated with gallstones include prolonged use of estrogen or progesterone, hypothyroidism, hepatitis, pancreatic disease, parasitic infestation, and obesity.

SUGGESTED READINGS

1. Jutras JA, Levesque HP: Adenomyoma and adenomyomatosis of the gallbladder. Radiol Clin North Am 4:483–500, 1966
2. Lasser EC: Pharmacodynamics of biliary contrast media. Radiol Clin North Am 4:511–519, 1966
3. Ochsner SF: Solitary polypoid lesions of the gallbladder. Radiol Clin North Am 4:501–510, 1966
4. Weens HS, Walker LA: The radiologic diagnosis of acute cholecystitis and pancreatitis. Radiol Clin North Am 2:89–106, 1964
5. Wise RE: Current concepts of intravenous cholangiography. Radiol Clin North Am 4:521–523, 1966

CORRECT ANSWERS

Question 80-(C)
Question 81-(E)
Question 82-(C)
Question 83-(C)
Question 84-(E)
Question 85-(E)

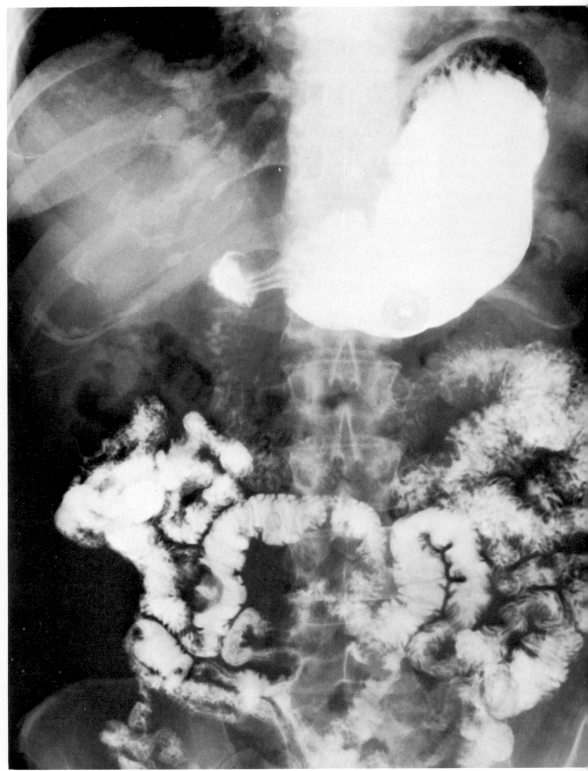

Figure 41. This 55-year-old woman has tarry stools and loss of appetite and weight. You are shown a roentgenogram taken during a small bowel examination.

Questions 86 and 87

86. Which one of the following is the *MOST* likely diagnosis?

    (A)   Metastatic melanoma
    (B)   Kaposi's sarcoma
    (C)   Leiomyosarcoma
    (D)   Lymphosarcoma
    (E)   Ectopic pancreas

87. Which one of the following neoplasms has the highest incidence in the ileum?

    (A)   Kaposi's sarcoma
    (B)   Leiomyosarcoma
    (C)   Fibrosarcoma
    (D)   Lymphosarcoma
    (E)   Adenocarcinoma

Discussion

QUESTION 86

Did you look carefully at Figure 41? If you did you saw several ulcerated lesions in the small bowel as well as one involving the stomach (indicated by *arrows* on Figure 41A). In addition, there are multiple nodules within the right lung base seen through the liver.

Because of their appearance these lesions have been called "bull's-eye lesions". Although not pathognomonic for metastatic melanoma, multiple nodules within the lungs and the intestinal tract, and their "bull's-eye" na-

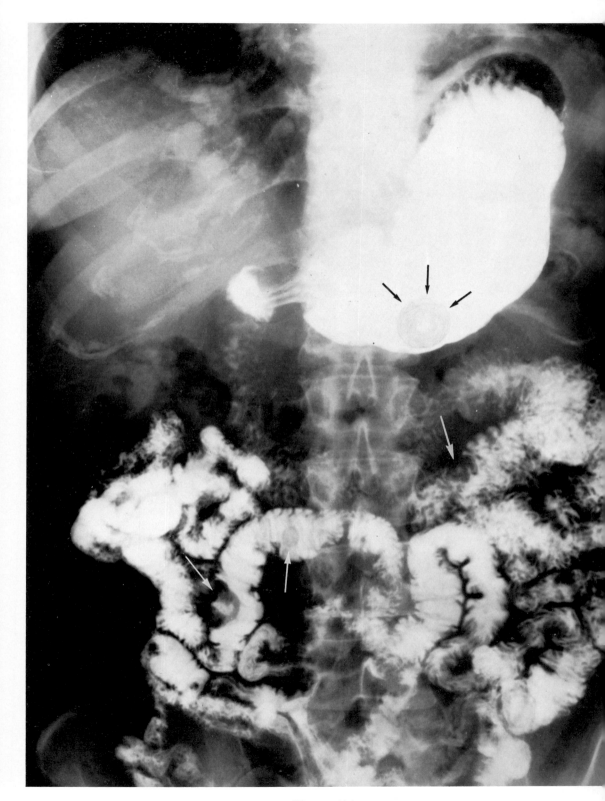

Figure 41A

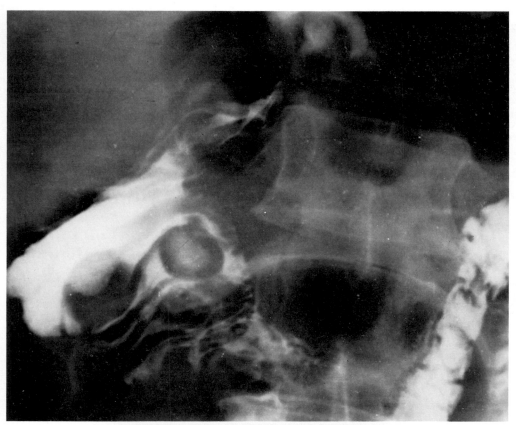

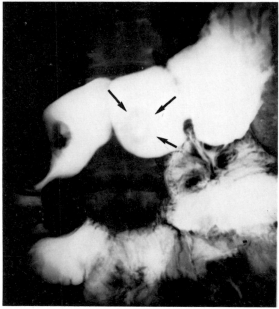

Figures 41B (top) and C (bottom)

ture, make **metastatic melanoma (A) the most likely diagnosis.** Figures 41B and C demonstrate "bull's-eye" lesions of malignant melanoma in two other patients (*arrows*).

Melanoma is one of the two most common lesions metastasizing to the gastrointestinal tract; the other is carcinoma of the breast. The most common primary sites of melanoma are, of course, the eye and the skin, although others including the female genitalia, the nervous system, the breast, and the anus have been described.

A few cases of primary lesions of the intestinal tract have been described; however, the absence of melanoblasts above the mucocutaneous junction of the anus raises doubt concerning the validity of this diagnosis.

The "bull's-eye" lesions represent intraluminal or intramural metastases which have ulcerated or are umbilicated. Other roentgen findings may be extrinsic pressure defects on the intestinal tract due to the widespread metastatic involvement and intussusception with the metastatic lesion serving as the lead mass.

"Bull's-eye" lesions can occur with other primary and metastatic lesions of the bowel. Single lesions have been described in spindle cell tumors, lymphosarcoma, aberrant pancreas, carcinoid, and granuloma with eosinophiles. Multiple lesions have also been seen with Kaposi's sarcoma and Hodgkin's disease. The multiplicity of the lesions in this patient should have excluded all of the other suggested diagnoses, except, perhaps, Kaposi's sarcoma.

Kaposi sarcoma is an unusual malignant lesion of slow evolution, common in Italian and Jewish men but also extremely common in certain parts of Africa where it makes up 10 per cent of all malignant neoplasms.

The condition usually begins as a solitary skin nodule, but subsequently they may be multiple. In addition, the disease has multiple foci of origin; autopsy has shown involvement of the gastrointestinal tract, lymph nodes, liver, and bone. Pulmonary lesions are unusual.

QUESTION 87

Your answer to question 87 should be lymphosarcoma (D).

Tumors of the small bowel are relatively infrequent considering the large area that can be involved. In 1947, in the United States, the maximum adjusted incidence was 1 per 100,000 population. Although the majority encountered at operation are malignant, autopsy shows that benign tumors occur most frequently. Of 327 malignant tumors reported in the small bowel, about 18 per cent were in the duodenum, 36 per cent in the jejunum, and 41 per cent in the ileum.

Adenocarcinoma is the most common malignant tumor of the small bowel, but the vast majority are either in the duodenum or the jejunum. Lymphosarcoma is the second most frequent malignant lesion of the small bowel and is most prevalent in the ileum, far exceeding the incidence of carcinoma in this area. Leiomyosarcoma and fibrosacroma are distinctly unusual lesions.

One neoplasm commonly seen in the ileum but not listed here is the carcinoid. Although most carcinoid tumors arise within the appendix, 85 per cent of those involving the small bowel are within the ileum.

SUGGESTED READINGS

1. MacDonald RA: A study of 356 carcinoids of the gastrointestinal tract; report of four new cases of the carcinoid syndrome. Am J Med *21:*867–878, 1956
2. Pagtalunan RJG, Mayo CW, Dockerty MG: Primary malignant tumors of the small intestine. Am J Surg *108:*13–18, 1964
3. Pomerantz H, Margolin HN: Metastases to the gastrointestinal tract from malignant melanoma. Am J Roentgenol *88:*712–717, 1962

CORRECT ANSWERS

Question 86-(A)
Question 87-(D)

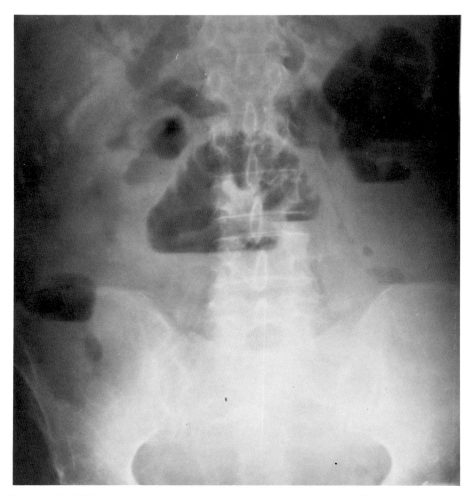

Figure 42. This 35-year-old woman has been vomiting. You are shown a roentgenogram of the abdomen taken with the patient in the upright position.

Questions 88 through 90

88. Which one of the following is the *MOST* likely diagnosis?

    (A)   Intussusception
    (B)   Small bowel obstruction due to adhesion
    (C)   Mesenteric infarction
    (D)   Appendicitis with ileus
    (E)   None of the above

89. Which one of the following statements about intussusception of the small intestine in adults is *MOST* likely?

    (A)   It is rarely associated with a lead mass
    (B)   It is most easily demonstrated with a retrograde barium study
    (C)   It is most often ileocolic
    (D)   It is most often acute in onset
    (E)   It is more often associated with a benign than with a malignant process

90. Which one of the following signs *MOST* strongly suggests mesenteric infarction in a patient with an acute abdomen?

    (A)   Dilatation of the small bowel and ascending and transverse colon
    (B)   Marked vascular calcification
    (C)   Fluid-filled loops
    (D)   A "sentinel" loop
    (E)   Linear gas shadows in the periphery of the liver

Discussion

QUESTION 88

Figure 42 demonstrates a dilated loop of small bowel with air-fluid levels in the mid abdomen. There is increased density in the lower portion of the abdomen, suggesting the presence of fluid or fluid-filled loops. Several short fluid levels are also seen in other loops of small bowel. Of primary interest is the branching, gas-filled structure within the right upper quadrant, representing air within the biliary tree. The findings, then, of gas within the biliary tree and mechanical small bowel obstruction are two of the three roentgen manifestations of gallstone ileus, although the third member of the triad, ectopic gallstone, is not demonstrated on this study. **The most likely answer to question 88 is (E) "None of the above",** since "gallstone ileus" was not offered as a possible answer.

The incidence of gallstone ileus varies from 0.4 to 5 per cent of all cases of small bowel obstruction. It is, of course, higher in the older age group and 80 per cent occur in women. Symptoms are essentially nonspecific, mimicking those of small bowel obstruction of any type, except there is often a previous history of gallbladder disease. The one clinical finding that may suggest gallstone ileus is a history of intermittent episodes of abdominal cramps, nausea, and vomiting occurring over several days. These symptoms are due to the intermittent obstructive nature of the stone as it passes through the bowel. The full-blown signs of bowel obstruction do not supervene until obturation occurs, usually in the ileum.

Although the roentgen triad of gallstone ileus in small bowel obstruction, internal biliary fistula, and ectopic gallstone, the presence of all three findings is unusual. In one series, 86 per cent of patients showed the obstructive pattern, 60 per cent had gas within the gallbladder or biliary tree, but in only 25 per cent was the calculus demonstrated.

Air in the biliary tree may be caused by many conditions other than a biliary fistula. These include infection by gas-forming organisms, after sphincterotomy, a patulous spincter of Oddi as seen in aged patients, or passage of a stone through the sphincter of Oddi. Therefore, this finding alone need not imply gallstone ileus. Of course, the gallstone may pass through the bowel without causing obstruction and, therefore, the combination of air in the biliary tree and an ectopic gallstone also does not always indicate gallstone ileus. *Obstruction* of the small bowel is a necessary concomitant.

In the presence of the triad, no further work-up is required. If only one or two of the triad is demonstrated, however, opaque contrast media may be helpful in confirming the diagnosis.

None of the other diagnoses listed in question 88 is associated with branching linear gas shadows within the right upper quadrant except mesenteric infarction. Gas in the portal vein as a result of mesenteric infarction has been well established. The differentiation, however, between biliary gas and portal venous gas is relatively easy. Although the portal vein and biliary radicals follow the same course within the liver, the centripetal flow of bile causes gas to be collected within the main duct system (as seen in Figure 42) and none to be in the periphery of the liver in gallstone ileus. On the other hand, the centrifugal flow of portal blood causes the venous gas to accumulate within the *periphery* (*arrows*, Figure 42A) of the liver rather than within the central portion. If sufficient portal venous gas is present, it may be seen in the more central radicals as well (Figures 42A and B), *lower arrows*).

QUESTION 89

Your answer to question 89 should have been (E) because (A) through (D) are more characteristic of intussusception in the pediatric than in the adult patient.

As opposed to infants and young children in which 95 per cent of intussusceptions are idiopathic, in adults 80 per cent have a specific cause. In a large series of adults with intussusception, a benign tumor was the etiology in one third and a malignant tumor in one fifth of the patients. In 22 per cent of the cases no cause was found. Unlike children in which only 4 per cent of the intussusceptions are confined to the small bowel, in adults 40 per cent of the intussusceptions are confined to the small bowel and only 29 per cent are ileocecal or ileocolic. Therefore, barium from above is far more accurate than a retrograde study in most cases. As opposed to the child in whom the onset is usually abrupt, intussusception in adults is characterized most often by chronic or subacute symptoms with irregular *recurring* episodes of colicky pain, nausea, and vomiting. You are referred to question 102, pp. 232–237, for a full discussion of this entity.

QUESTION 90

As mentioned previously, **linear gas shadows in the periphery of the liver (E)** representing portal venous gas are highly suggestive of mesenteric infarction. Such shadows have been described in acute hemorrhagic enterocolitis in childhood (see Figures 30, 30A and B), following hydrogen peroxide enema, in necrosis of the bowel from nonvascular causes, and in just marked gaseous distention of the intestine. When noted, a careful study for gas in venous radicals of the bowel should be made (Figure 42C). Although

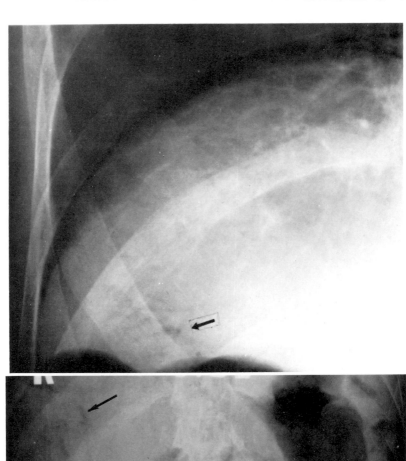

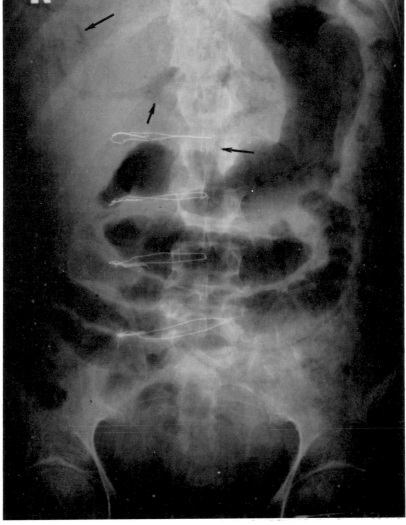

Figures 42A (top) and B (bottom)

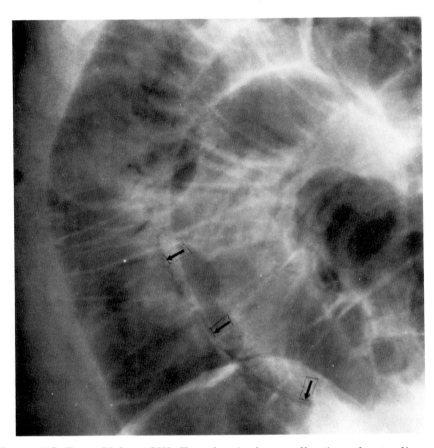

Figure 42C From Nelson SW: Extraluminal gas collections due to diseases of the gastrointestinal tract. Am J Roentgenol *115*:225–248, 1972 (with permission of the author and publisher).

answers (A) through (D) may occur with mesenteric infarction, they are in no way diagnostic nor nearly as suggestive of this diagnosis as answer (E). Dilatation of the small bowel and ascending and transverse colon are occasionally seen with mesenteric infarction since this is the vascular distribution of the superior mesenteric artery. However, other diseases such as carcinoma of the splenic flexure may result in a similar pattern. Fluid-filled loops, again an occasional manifestation of mesenteric infarction, also occur in other acute abdominal conditions. A "sentinel" loop, although sometimes seen with mesenteric infarction, is more suggestive of a localized inflammatory reaction.

SUGGESTED READINGS

1. Eisenman JI, Finck EJ, O'Loughlin BJ: Gallstone ileus. A review of the roentgenographic findings and report of a new roentgen sign. Am J Roentgencl *101:*361–366, 1967
2. Nelson SW: Extraluminal gas collections due to diseases of the gastrointestinal tract. Am J Roentgenol *115:*225–248, 1972

CORRECT ANSWERS

Question 88-(E)
Question 89-(E)
Question 90-(E)

NOTES

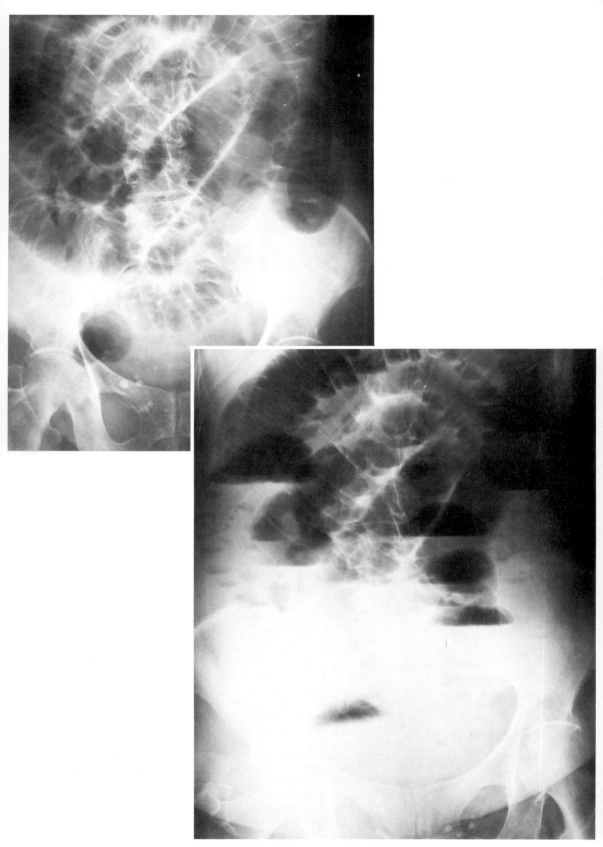

Figures 43 (top) and 44 (bottom). This 72-year-old woman complains of abdominal pain. Roentgenograms of the abdomen were taken with the patient in the supine (Figure 43) and upright (Figure 44) positions.

Questions 91 through 93

91. Which one of the following is the *MOST* likely diagnosis?

   (A) Paralytic ileus
   (B) Gallstone ileus
   (C) Obstruction of the small bowel
   (D) Pseudo-obstruction of the small bowel
   (E) Vascular occlusion

92. Which one of the following conditions is *LEAST* likely to be associated with ischemic necrosis of the bowel?

   (A) Intussusception
   (B) Volvulus
   (C) Gallstone ileus
   (D) Obstruction due to adhesion
   (E) Incarcerated hernia

93. Which one of the following is *LEAST* characteristic of mechanical obstruction of the small intestine?

   (A) Long air-fluid levels
   (B) "Step-ladder" pattern of distended loops
   (C) Separation of loops
   (D) Absence of gas in the colon
   (E) Dilated fluid-filled loops

Discussion

QUESTION 91

Figure 43 demonstrates multiple, dilated, air-filled loops of small bowel and a hernia in the right lower quadrant as manifested by a small part of a gas-containing loop of small intestine which extends below the expected location of the right inguinal ligament. On the radiograph this gas-containing loop appears just above and medial to the right femoral head. In Figure 44, an upright film, there are multiple air-fluid levels and an increased density within the pelvis, indicating fluid-filled loops. This combination of findings and the presence of the Richter's type of hernia make **obstruction of the small bowel (C) the most likely diagnosis of those listed in question 91.**

The lack of distention of the colon lessens the probability of paralytic ileus as the diagnosis, although occasionally (particularly in the postoperative patient) dilatation confined to the small bowel may result in paralytic ileus simulating small bowel obstruction.

A diagnosis of gallstone ileus cannot be made in this patient because only obstruction is present; the other two criteria of gallstone ileus—an aberrant gallstone and gas within the biliary system—are not seen.

Pseudo-obstruction of the small intestine is an uncommon condition but one in which the roentgen and clinical manifestations closely mimic those of obstruction. It is not likely to be associated with hernia, however. It may be divided into three forms: (1) transient pseudo-obstruction associated with electrolyte imbalance, renal failure, congestive failure, and other acute problems; (2) chronic pseudo-obstruction as seen with multiple chronic systemic diseases, including scleroderma and amyloidosis; and (3) idiopathic pseudo-obstruction, a condition not associated with other disease and almost invariably seen in young women.

A vascular occlusion could produce all of the findings seen here except that of the Richter's type of hernia, which, when recognized, establishes the mechanical nature of the obstruction and precludes the other possibilities listed here.

QUESTION 92

Intussusception, volvulus, gallstone ileus, and incarcerated hernia can all cause vascular compromise and resulting ischemic necrosis. **Simple obstruction due to adhesion (D),** on the other hand, except when associated with a so-called closed-loop obstruction, is not associated with vascular compromise.

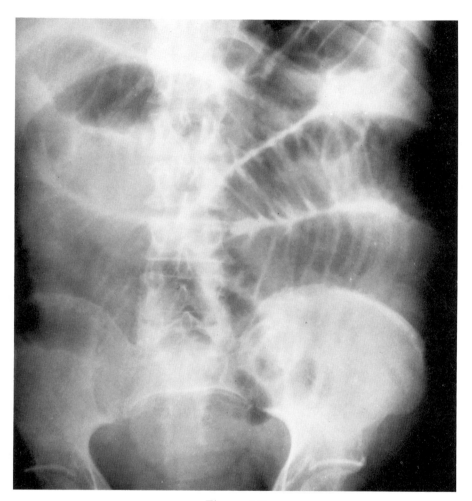

Figure 44A

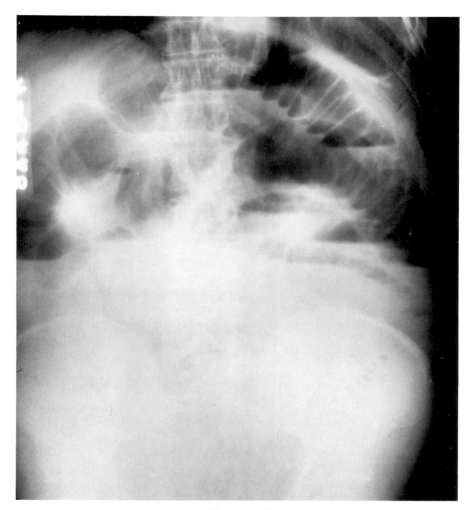

Figure 44B

QUESTION 93

In question 93 all of the listed answers are characteristic of mechanical obstruction of the small bowel. However, **separation of loops, (C) is only** a very late manifestation and when present is secondary to edema of the wall or the development of peritonitis due to the long-standing nature of the obstruction.

Although absence of gas in the colon with small bowel distention is one of the findings in small bowel obstruction, special mention must be made of the occasional finding of only small bowel dilatation (Figures 44A and B) in the presence of colon obstruction (Figure 44C). Because of this and the

216 / *Gastrointestinal Tract Disease*

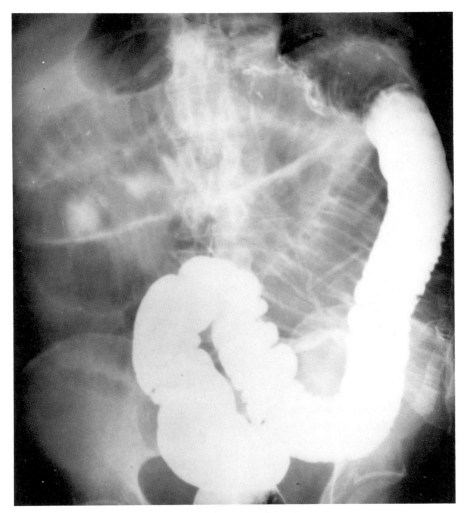

Figure 44C

danger of barium impaction proximal to such a colon obstruction a barium enema should be done before barium is given by mouth. This procedure showed an obstruction in the splenic flexure (Figure 44C).

SUGGESTED READINGS

1. Frimann-Dahl J: *Roentgen Examinations in Acute Abdominal Diseases.* Charles C Thomas, Springfield, Ill, 1960
2. Moss AA, Goldberg HI, Brotman M: Idiopathic intestinal pseudo-obstruction. Am J Roentgenol *115*:312–317, 1972

CORRECT ANSWERS
Question 91-(C)
Question 92-(D)
Question 93-(C)

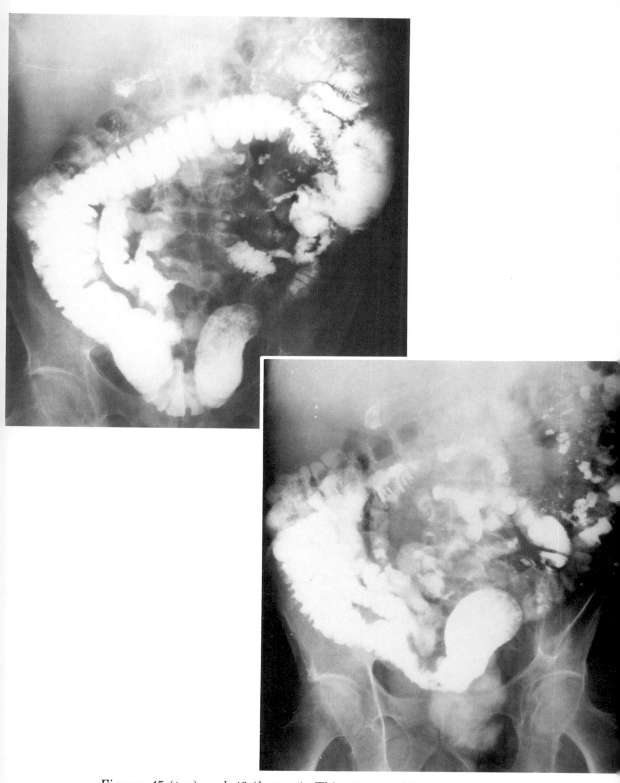

Figures 45 (top) and 46 (bottom). This 71-year-old man was admitted in congestive failure. He has had cramping mid abdominal pain with occasional nausea and vomiting for 4 months. Roentgenograms of the abdomen were taken with the patient in the prone position at 2 hours (Figure 45) and 4 hours (Figure 46) after the oral ingestion of barium sulfate.

Questions 94 through 97

94. Which one of the following is the *MOST* likely diagnosis?

    (A) Carcinoma
    (B) Intussusception
    (C) Meckel's diverticulum
    (D) Stricture
    (E) Gallstone ileus

95. Intussusception in the adult is *MOST* commonly due to

    (A) Meckel's diverticulum
    (B) benign small bowel tumor
    (C) malignant small bowel tumor
    (D) lymphoid hyperplasia
    (E) adhesions

96. Which one of the following is the *DEFINITIVE* diagnostic sign of gallstone ileus?

    (A) Gas in the biliary ducts
    (B) Small bowel obstruction
    (C) Annular calcification within the abdomen
    (D) Air-fluid levels in the gallbladder
    (E) None of the above

97. Which one of the following complications of Meckel's diverticulum is *LEAST* common?

    (A) Intestinal obstruction
    (B) Peptic ulcer
    (C) Bleeding
    (D) Perforation
    (E) Calcified enteroliths

Discussion

Figures 45 and 46 demonstrate incomplete small bowel obstruction secondary to **stricture (D).**

Although all of the answers listed in question 94 can be responsible for small bowel obstruction, the history of 4 months of symptoms suggests some chronic condition. This virtually excludes intussusception, Meckel's diverticulum, and gallstone ileus since these are relatively acute problems (although any may occasionally have intermittent obstructive symptoms for several days). Intussusception is also excluded because of the absence of the roentgenologic criteria described on p. 233 in this syllabus. This leaves carcinoma and stricture as the most probable causes of the obstruction.

As you note, the end of the obstructed segment is smooth and club-shaped, and there is a very short transition area between the dilated and the collapsed segment. In carcinoma, the transition between the dilated and collapsed normal bowel is generally longer and the dilated segment is irregular due to encroachment of the tumor.

Obstruction secondary to an adhesion would give a similar appearance to the stricture seen here.

This man, as stated in the clinical information, was admitted in congestive failure. He had received supplemental potassium therapy for 10 months prior to admission and the stricture demonstrated here was potassium induced (Figure 46A).

The relationship of ulcers and stenosis to potassium therapy is well known. From experimental as well as clinical evidence, it appears that the ulcer and stricture are on the basis of vascular changes. These changes involve arteries, veins, and lymphatics (both mesenteric and intramural), and simulate closely the vascular alterations seen in Crohn's disease as well as those seen with ulcerative colitis. Segmental or concentric intimal thickening, with marked luminal compromise of the involved vessels, are the pathologic findings.

Figure 46A shows the segment of resected bowel. The stenosis (*arrows*) is short and the ulcer is still active. In Figure 46B, another patient, the ulcer has healed leaving only the stricture (*arrows*).

QUESTION 95

All of the conditions listed in question 95 can evoke intussusception in the adult. However, **benign small bowel tumor (B)** comprises one third of the

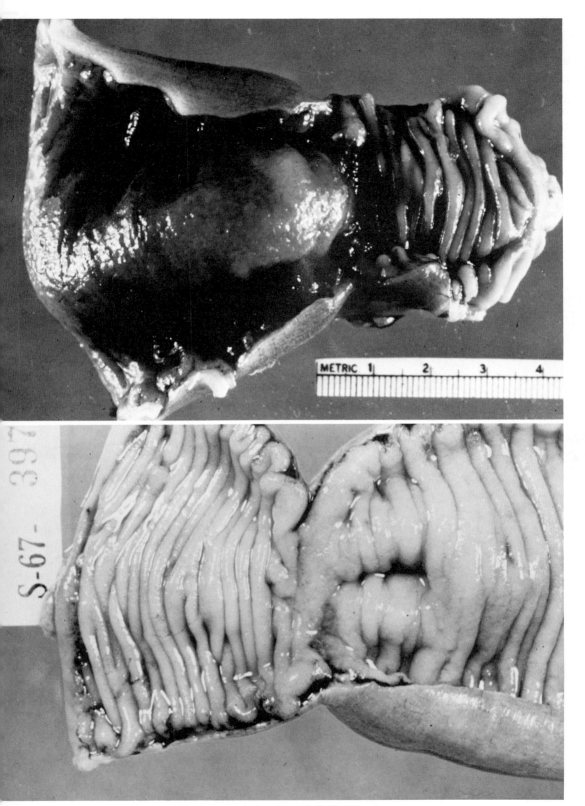

Figures 46A (top) and B (bottom)

cases and far exceeds all other causes. Other causes include malignant tumors in a fifth of the patients, and infrequently Meckel's diverticulum, chronic ulcer, adhesions and bands, aberrant pancreas, and foreign body. It must be pointed out, however, that in 22 per cent of the patients no cause is found for the intussusception. In children, lymphoid hyperplasia is the most common cause although lymphoma must also be suspected in the older child.

QUESTION 96

In question 96 all of the listed answers can be seen in gallstone ileus. However, none is definitive *alone*. **The correct answer to question 96 then is (E), none of the above.** Answers (A), (B), and (C) represent the triad which when present is diagnostic of gallstone ileus. Since, however, in only 25 per cent of patients with gallstone ileus is the gallstone actually demonstrated, the chance of having these three signs present is not great. Although air-fluid levels in the gallbladder may be a concomitant of gallstone ileus, they seem to be much more prevalent in emphysematous cholecystitis.

QUESTION 97

In question 97 all of the listed complications are seen with Meckel's diverticulum. In children the most common symptom of Meckel's diverticulum is bleeding, almost invariably secondary to aberrant gastric mucosa with resulting ulceration. In adults, intestinal obstruction is the most common symptom. This obstruction may be due to volvulus, inflammation, and adhesions, or to invagination and intussusception. It should be pointed out, however, that in a large series of Meckel's diverticula reported in 1962, 560 of 722 were found as incident findings either at surgery or autopsy. Complications included intussusception in 15, inflammation in 29, obstruction other than intussusception in 28, hemorrhage in 63, and neoplasm in 10.

Calcified enteroliths within Meckel's diverticulum are well-known entities. Their radiographic demonstration, however, is much less common than their actual incidence. and they are often confused with appendiceal calculi or even gallstones. Perforation as a complication of Meckel's diverticulum is quite *rare*. In a series of 722 cases this complication was not described. **The answer to Question 97 is** therefore **(D), perforation.**

SUGGESTED READINGS

1. Boley SJ: *Vascular Disorders of the Intestine.* Appleton-Century-Crofts, New York, 1971
2. Christiansen KH, Cancelmo RP: Meckel's stone ileus. Am J Roentgenol 99: 139–141, 1967

3. Nelson SW, Christoforidis AJ: The use of barium sulfate suspensions in the study of suspected mechanical obstruction of the small intestine. Am J Roentgenol *101:*367–378, 1967
4. Schwartz S, Boley S, Schultz L, Allen A: A survey of vascular diseases of the small intestine. Semin in Roentgenol *1:*178–218, 1966
5. Wiot JF, Spitz, HB: Small bowel intussusception demonstrated by oral barium. Radiology *97:*361–366, 1970

CORRECT ANSWERS

Question 94-(D)
Question 95-(B)
Question 96-(E)
Question 97-(D)

NOTES

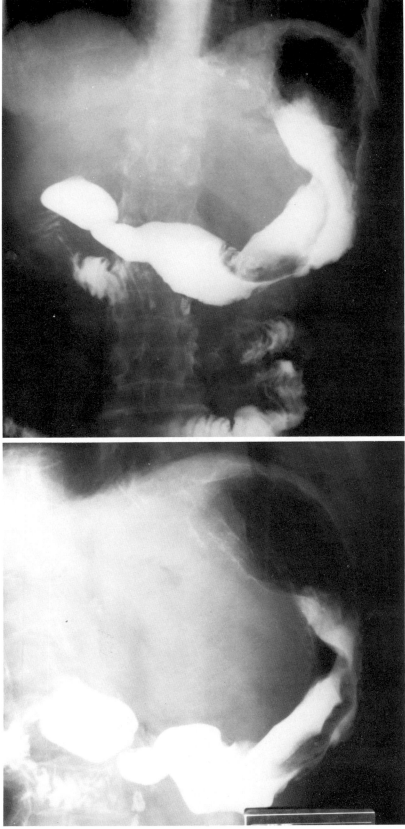

Figures 47 (top) and 48 (bottom). This 63-year-old woman has a 7-month history of epigastric pain and weight loss. You are shown two roentgenograms of the stomach.

Questions 98 through 101

98. Which one of the following is the *MOST* likely diagnosis?

    (A)   Malignant ulcer
    (B)   Benign ulcer
    (C)   Retrogastric mass
    (D)   Intramural mass
    (E)   Ectopic pancreas

99. Which one of the following roentgenographic findings is *MOST* suggestive of a malignant gastric ulcer?

    (A)   Penetration beyond the wall of the stomach
    (B)   An ulcer greater than 3 cm. in diameter
    (C)   A profiled ulcer which lies within the lumen
    (D)   Abrupt transition between normal mucosa and the soft tissue mound surrounding the crater
    (E)   Folds radiating into the crater

100. Which one of the following statements about gastric ulcers is *CORRECT*?

    (A)   Ulcers which become larger during therapy are malignant
    (B)   Ulcers which become smaller during therapy are benign
    (C)   Ulcers on the greater curvature are usually malignant
    (D)   Gastric ulcers should be considered malignant and treated surgically
    (E)   None of the above

101. Which one of the following statements concerning leiomyomas is *IN-CORRECT*?

    (A)   The roentgenographic differential diagnosis from leiomyosarcomas is usually impossible
    (B)   Ulceration and mucosal bleeding are characteristic
    (C)   They are less common in the stomach than in any other part of the gastrointestinal tract
    (D)   They may contain calcification
    (E)   They usually show the roentgenographic features of submucosal tumors

Discussion

This lesion is typical for a large ulcerated neoplasm with rolled, elevated edges (A). The lesion is seen in profile, the ulcer crater therefore appears as a barium collection between the opposed (anterior and posterior) walls. The elevated margins of the tumor trap a semicircular collection of barium. In this case, the patient is lying in the prone position. This compresses the stomach in the AP position and approximates the rolled edges of the tumor crater. The base or floor of the crater is the ulcerated surface of the gastric wall which lies in its expected position (Figure 47A, "A" *arrows*), and is not much thicker than the normal gastric wall would be. This is because the tumor tissue in this area has become necrotic and the remainder of the tumor in the gastric wall has elicited a fibrotic response which maintains the integrity of the lumen at that point. However, there is a large rolled edge of tumor (Figure 47A, "B" *arrows*) around the margins of the crater where the neoplasm is close to the blood supply in the adjacent normal portions of the stomach. When such a crater is compressed by the examiner, or as in this case by the patient lying in the prone position, it will have an appearance in which the outer part of the trapped barium collection will be just about where the normal gastric lumen would be expected to be. The border of the barium collection facing the lumen is inward convex. This shape results from the opposed anterior and posterior portions of the elevated edge of the tumor, the barium being trapped much as it would be if one folded the cap of a soft drink bottle. Note the nodularity of the margin of this rim of tumor tissue where it is contiguous to the normal gastric lumen (Figure 48A, "C" *arrows*). These films show the characteristic abrupt transition between the normal lesser curvature and the point where it meets the edge of the tumor (Figure 47A, "D" *arrows*). This is highly suggestive of neoplasm as opposed to the gradual smooth transition between normal gastric wall and the mound of edema which surrounds benign craters (B). (See discussion of benign and malignant ulcers on pp. 30–39 with particular reference to Carman's sign as depicted in Figures 6-O, P, and Q.)

The *intraluminal* location of a large crater, which when seen tangentially, has a sharply defined convex margin facing the gastric lumen, is not the configuration seen in large benign ulcers. Benign ulcers can be surrounded by large zones of edema which can cause diagnostic problems but rarely does one find in benign disease the nodularity seen here. A retrogastric mass

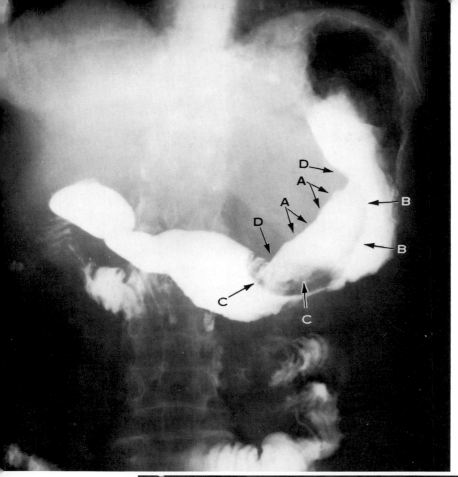

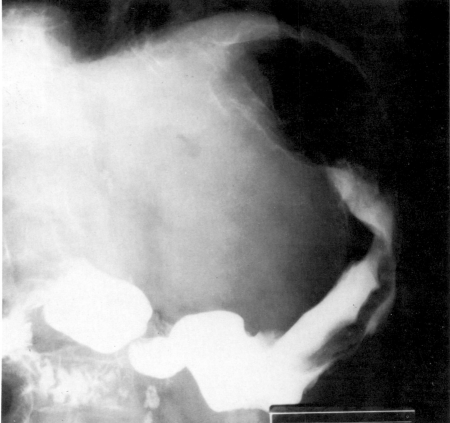

Figures 47A (top) and B (bottom)

(C) may produce a semicircular thinned area in the intragastric barium, but the *loss of density* will *increase* going toward the edge of the stomach on frontal films and the distinct rolled edge will be absent. Some element of retrogastric mass could be present in this case due to retrogastric lymph node masses, but the appearance of the lesion on the presented films is primarily due to the described apposition of the rolled edges of the *gastric* lesion.

Intramural masses (D) cause smooth, roundish lumps protruding toward the lumen. The transition zone may be quite sharp and ulcers may occur in these masses. Scirrhous carcinoma of the stomach produces a diffuse thickening of the wall, and is not characterized by intraluminal elevated components as seen here; furthermore, scirrhous carcinomas are rather subtle because of the rather diffuse narrowing and the lack of intraluminal masses.

Ectopic pancreas (E) is not at all a good suggestion, since the lesion is *much* larger than the average ectopic pancreas (most are less than 2 cm. in diameter), the ulceration is huge (compared to the small central dimple seen in ectopic pancreas) and the lesser curvature is not a common location for ectopic pancreas (most occur in the *duodenum* or *distal* stomach).

QUESTION 99

Abrupt transition between normal mucosa and the soft tissue mound surrounding the crater (D) is the correct answer. Many carcinomas arise from the surface epithelium. Hence, as the growth progresses, there will be a sharp transition from normal to abnormal. This to some extent is also due to the globular type of growth associated with many tumors. This sharp transition point is rather characteristic of tumor and serves as an excellent differential diagnostic point. However, it should be remembered that certain tumors infiltrate under the mucosa and, therefore, will cause a *gradual* constriction of the lumen. This may occur in some carcinomas of the esophagus where the constriction may occasionally be a gentle one rather than an abrupt one, in scirrhous carcinoma of the stomach and in what is sometimes known as scirrhous carcinoma of the colon. Penetration beyond the wall of the stomach (A) is a characteristic sign of benign ulceration. The size of the ulcer crater (B) is of no consequence. While in past years it has been said that ulcers over 4 cm. (or other numbers as given by each author) are characteristically malignant, this is not so. One encounters now and then huge benign craters. Intraluminal location (C) is generally a good sign for malignancy. However, with marked swelling and with incomplete distention of the stomach, it is frequently hard to demonstrate penetration in cases of benign ulcers and, therefore, this sign is not as reliable as the abrupt transition sign (D). Radiating folds (E) may be encountered both with malignant and benign craters. It is helpful to try to analyze the nature and appearance of the folds. If the folds are smooth, slender, and actually extend into the edge of the crater, the lesion is most likely benign. If the folds are somewhat irregular in shape and if they merge into a mound of polypoid tissue around the crater, the lesion is likely to be malignant. Again, the diagnostic value is not as great as that of the abrupt transition sign.

QUESTION 100

The correct answer to this question is (E). While it is true that ulcers which heal rapidly are more likely to be benign, and those which don't heal are more likely malignant, observations show that malignant ulcers can heal partially, and, rarely, even completely, only for the lesion to become apparent again some months later. This has been shown in the Japanese studies of carcinoma growth patterns. These months, of course, represent wasted possible treatment time. Increase in the size of the ulceration during treatment (A) is a better sign of malignancy but also is not absolute since even in the cases of benign ulcers multiple factors may influence the size of the crater and its behavior. The curvature location (C) is of no great significance. While this statement about the greater curvature has been made in the past, it really is not very helpful as a differential diagnostic aid. (D) is not particularly applicable. At present a great majority of gastric ulcers in this country (over 90 per cent) are benign. Most of them will heal on medical treatment. There is some dissenting surgical opinion on this. However, even if treated surgically, the treatment for a gastric carcinoma and a benign gastric ulcer is different and it is helpful to know the diagnosis before surgery.

QUESTION 101

All of these statements are true descriptions of leiomyomas except for **(C)—leiomyoma *is* a *common* tumor of the stomach.** To comment on the other answers: (A) while the classical benign leiomyoma is a round smooth tumor, frequently with a central ulceration, and the leiomyosarcoma a bulky, frequently lobulated mass with a large, frequently irregular ulceration, the actual differential diagnosis between malignant and benign lesion is quite difficult to make, even at the time of histological study of the lesion. Sometimes it is almost necessary to determine the subsequent course of events to make this decision, although most of the time histology is a satisfactory method of differential diagnosis. (B) ulceration is indeed quite characteristic, as is bleeding. Bleeding may be a common first manifestation of a gastric leiomyoma since the lesion itself is rather painless. (D) calcification may occur, although it is unusual. (E) the lesion arises in the muscular layers of the stomach and thus appears as a classical intramural mass, frequently protruding extensively toward the stomach and being covered by a smooth layer of stretched mucosa which, however, may ulcerate.

DISCUSSION

Much about the criteria of diagnosis has been said in the above. The question arises: is it of any consequence to make this differentiation? Indeed, it is of some consequence. Surgical treatment differs for the two types of lesions and a great deal of time, suffering, and, possibly, life could be saved if early accurate diagnosis could be achieved. Improved endoscopic diagnosis is now possible with the flexible fiberoptic gastroscope which has been a significant addition to the diagnostic capabilities of the gastroenterologist. In turn, his observations will help establish more reliable radiological diagnostic criteria and thus contribute to our ability in diagnosis. The relative simplicity of an upper gastrointestinal roentgen examination (as compared with endoscopic study), and the great frequency with which these are done, mandates that an attempt should be made to establish as accurate a diagnosis as possible to the extent it is objectively justifiable.

The radiologist who identifies an ulcer crater in the stomach should make an attempt to separate these lesions into either (a) clearly benign, (b) clearly malignant, or (c) indeterminate. Two review articles on the differential diagnosis of gastric ulcerations, namely the ones by Nelson and by Wolf, are very helpful and highly recommended. As Wolf states, the emphasis in the differential diagnostic efforts should be on *positive* signs rather than on the absence of certain other signs. The issue is made more difficult by the fact that not all carcinomas grow in the same way and, therefore, do not ulcerate in the same way. The ulceration in a large roundish mass may be very well defined and localized, yet ragged. In a spreading carcinoma, there may be a large flat depressed area with somewhat elevated edges. In a highly necrotic tumor, there may be a rather deep hole. In turn, in the case of benign ulcers, in some cases there is very extensive fibrotic induration in and around the crater with marked elevation of portions of the gastric wall and sometimes a surprising amount of rigidity. In these situations it may be quite appropriate to call the lesion indeterminate and let the final diagnosis be made by appropriate endoscopic or surgical means.

Lastly, a question might arise about the importance of early and frequent roentgen gastrointestinal examinations, especially in view of the now rapid spread of endoscopic study. There is no question that endoscopy has enabled one to obtain the diagnosis of lesions such as superficial erosive gastritis, which may lead to massive bleeding and yet may be exceedingly hard to diagnose by roentgen means. On the other hand, there are many different lesions of the stomach that are still easily missed by the gastroscope. In many of them very helpful roentgen examinations can be obtained. Considering the serious consequences in terms of suffering, complications, and possible risk of life, we see no alternative but to continue vigorous application of multiple diagnostic studies in the patient with gastric complaints and ensure careful application of diagnostic criteria.

SUGGESTED READINGS

1. Boldero JL, Lumsden K: The meniscus sign in ulcerating gastric carcinoma. J Fac Radiol 10:80–85, 1959
2. Carman RD: A new roentgen-ray sign of ulcerating gastric cancer. JAMA 77: 990–992, 1921
3. Jordan S: Gastric ulcer and cancer. Gastroenterology 34:254–268, 1958
4. Kirsch, IE: Roentgen diagnosability of gastric ulcer. A review of 100 proved cases of carcinoma of the stomach. Gastroenterology 37:53–59, 1959
5. Monafo WW Jr: Carcinoma of the stomach. Arch Surg 85:754–763, 1962
6. Nelson SW: A crescent-shaped collection of residual cholecystographic contrast material. A new sign of benign gastric ulcer? Am J Roentgenol 116: 293–303, 1972
7. Nelson SW: Discovery and differential diagnosis of gastric ulcers. Radiol Clin North Am 7:5–25, 1969
8. Palmer WL, Humphreys EM: Gastric Carcinoma: observations on peptic ulceration and healing. Gastroenterology 3:257–272, 1944
9. Palumbo LT, Sharpe WS: Gastric ulcer: is it benign or malignant? Arch Surg 85:705–710, 1962
10. Sakita T, Oguro Y, Takasu S, Fukutomi H, Miwa T, Yoshimori M: Observations on the healing of ulcerations in early gastric cancer. The life cycle of the malignant ulcer. Gastroenterology 60:835–844, 1971
11. Samuel E: Early diagnosis of gastric cancer. CRC Crit Rev Radiol Sci 3: 244–252, 1972
12. Strandjord NM, Moseley RD Jr, Schweinefus RL: Gastric carcinoma: accuracy of radiologic diagnosis. Radiology 74:442–451, 1960
13. Templeton FE: The gastric ulcer—benign or malignant? Editorial. Gastroenterology 37:109–110, 1959
14. Wolf BS: Observations on roentgen features of benign and malignant gastric ulcers. Simin in Roentgenol 6: 140–150, 1971

CORRECT ANSWERS

Question 98-(A)
Question 99-(D)
Question 100-(E)
Question 101-(C)

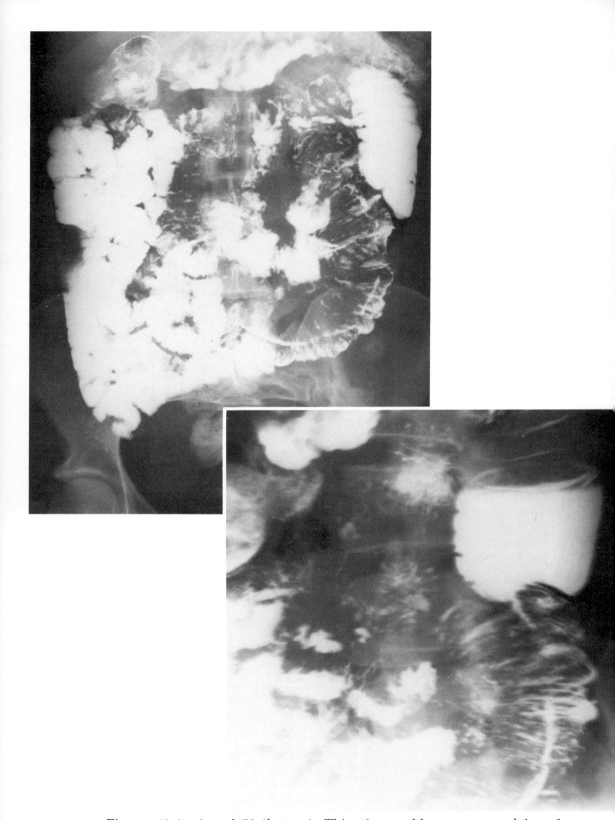

Figures 49 (top) and 50 (bottom). This 40-year-old woman complains of intermittent vomiting and epigastric pain. Figure 49 is a roentgenogram taken 2 hours after oral ingestion of barium sulfate, and Figure 50 is a spot roentgenogram taken shortly afterwards with the patient in the upright position.

Question 102

102. Which one of the following is the *MOST* likely diagnosis?

    (A)   Carcinoma of the jejunum
    (B)   Lymphoma of the jejunum
    (C)   Intussusception
    (D)   Regional enteritis
    (E)   Gallstone ileus

Discussion

The small bowel series films in Figures 49 and 50 demonstrate incomplete obstruction of the jejunum secondary to **intussusception (C).** The roentgen manifestations of intussusception of the small bowel using contrast media from above are characteristic but differ somewhat from those demonstrated by barium enema.

Schatzki, in his classic description of the roentgen findings of intussusception shown by barium enema, defined three concentric cylinders at the intussusception site (Figure 50A): (1) a central canal, (2) a peripheral sheath separated by (3) a space which contains the intussuscepted mesentery lined by the serosa of the two telescoped intestinal segments. Barium enema reveals the distal end of the intussusceptum as a cup-shaped filling defect. Often a tumor mass is seen as an added filling defect. Barium in the peripheral sheath outlines the circular bands of crowded haustra in the intussuscipiens resulting in a spiral or coiled spring appearance. Occasionally the central canal of the intussusceptum is seen.

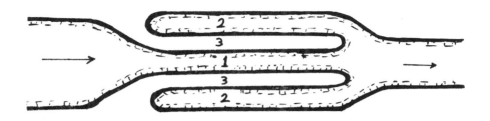

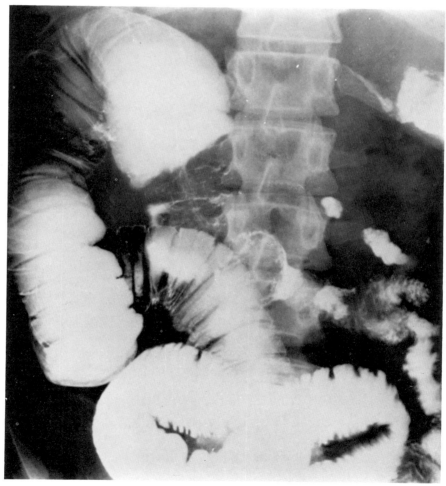

Figures 50A (top) and B (bottom)

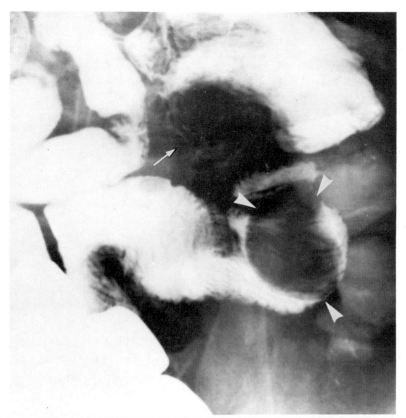

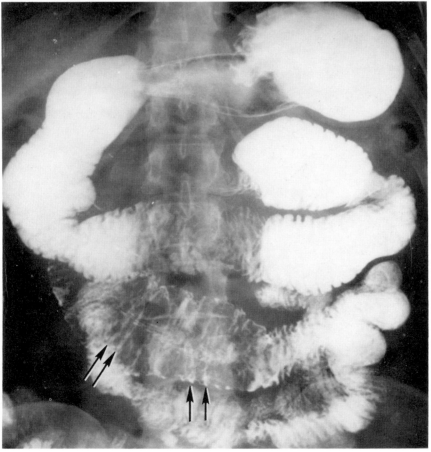

Figures 50C (top) and D (bottom)

In this patient the proximal small intestine is grossly distended. There is a sudden beak-like change in caliber at the site of the obstruction, at the level of vertebral body L1 in Figure 50B, as the central canal of the intussusceptum fills (Figure 50B). With incomplete obstruction, the central canal may be long, and longitudinal folds are often seen within it as we note in our case. Once the barium passes through the central canal it enters the normal bowel distal to the lesion. A lead mass, if present, can often be demonstrated. It is partially obscured in our case but can be seen exactly overlying the interspace between vertebral bodies L2 and L3 in Figure 50B. In Figure 50C an inverted Meckel's diverticulum serves as the lead mass (*arrowheads*). Longitudinal folds in the central canal are faintly seen (*arrow*). If barium passes retrograde into the intussuscipiens the coiled spring pattern is observed (Figure 50D, *arrows*).

With intussusception the mesentery is pulled forward and caught between the overlapping layers of bowel often causing vascular compression with compromise of circulation to the gut. The bowel wall then becomes edematous, and blood and serum exude from the mucosa into the lumen and from the serosa resulting in adhesions which prevent spontaneous reduction of the intussusception. Gangrene with its attendant complications may ensue.

The hallmarks of intussusception are the demonstration of the central canal and the coiled spring pattern. Rarely, edema is so severe that there is complete obstruction of the central canal and the cause of the small intestinal obstruction cannot be distinguished roentgenologically.

About 90 per cent of intussusceptions in infants and children are idiopathic; whereas in the adult, about 80 per cent have a specific cause. Generally in adults a lead mass is present (Figure 50B). Such lead masses include benign and malignant tumors, inverted Meckel's diverticula (Figure 50C), and foreign body. Other causes are prolapsed mucosa, chronic ulcer, adhesions and bands, aberrant pancreas, trauma, and foreign body, including intestinal tubes.

Only 5 to 7 per cent of all intussusceptions occur in adults. In 40 per cent of these, the intussusception is confined to the small bowel as opposed to 4 per cent in infants. Unlike infants, adults often present with chronic or subacute symptoms: nausea, vomiting, and irregularly recurring episodes of colicky pain, and occasionally an abdominal mass. Abdominal tenderness, rigidity, and melena are uncommon. The intermittent character of symptoms probably results from spontaneous reduction and recurrence.

SUGGESTED READINGS

1. Good CA: Entero-enteric intussusception. Radiology *42*:122–127, 1944

2. Nelson SW, Christoforidis AJ: The use of barium sulfate suspensions in the study of suspected mechanical obstruction of the small intestine. Am J Roentgenol *101:*367–378, 1967
3. Schatzki R: The roentgenologic appearance of intussuscepted tumors of the colon, with and without barium examination. Am J Roentgenol *41:*549–563, 1939
4. Wiot JF, Spitz HB: Small bowel intussusception demonstrated by oral barium. Radiology *97:*361–366, 1970

CORRECT ANSWER

Question 102-(C)

NOTES

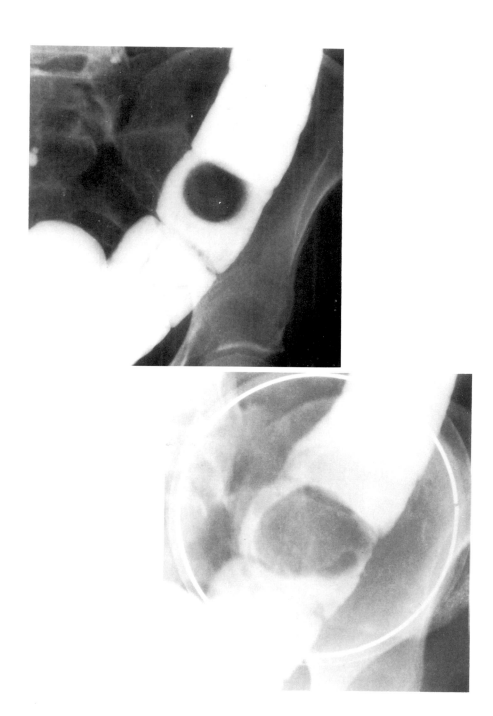

Figures 51 (top) and 52 (bottom). This 42-year-old woman has vague lowe abdominal distress. Figure 51 is a spot roentgenogram of the filled descend ing colon, and Figure 52 is a compression spot roentgenogram.

Questions 103 through 106

103. Which one of the following is the *MOST* likely diagnosis?

   (A)   Leiomyoma
   (B)   Villous adenoma
   (C)   Endometriosis
   (D)   Adenomatous polyp
   (E)   Lipoma

104. Which one of the following is *MOST* characteristic of villous adenoma?

   (A)   Multiple separate lesions
   (B)   Marked radiolucency
   (C)   Copious mucous secretions
   (D)   A smooth surface
   (E)   Most commonly found in the small intestine

105. Which one of the following statements concerning endometriosis is *LEAST* likely?

   (A)   It may cause obstruction
   (B)   Its most common intestinal location is the colon
   (C)   It appears as an intramural mass
   (D)   It is not usually associated with symptoms
   (E)   The lesions may be multiple

106. Which one of the following is the *MOST* common location of lipomas?

   (A)   Esophagus
   (B)   Stomach
   (C)   Duodenum
   (D)   Jejunum and ileum
   (E)   Colon

Discussion

QUESTION 103

The correct diagnosis in this case is lipoma (E). The roentgeno-grams show a very smoothly outlined, strikingly radiolucent round lesion (it appears even more radiolucent than the soft tissue density just outside the colon). The compression spot roentgenogram (Figure 52) shows the lesion to become larger. This is not simply due to projection. One can see that the lesion is larger even compared to the adjacent iliac bone. This rather clearly indicates that the lesion is *soft* and can be flattened by virtue of pressure. Villous adenoma (B) is not likely here because of the very smooth surface of the lesion. Characteristically, the villous adenoma is a frond-covered structure which has a rather streaky surface. The location would be quite favorable for villous adenoma. Endometriosis (C) is less likely because of the very clear intraluminal location of the mass (as indicated by the strikingly sharp definition of the contours of the lesion on Figure 51). Endometriosis arises from implantation of endometrial material on the outside of the bowel. Eventually this forms a cyst-like structure which is primarily intramural. As time goes on, considerable tissue reaction develops and there may be additional distortion and contraction of the segments of bowel involved. Leiomyoma (A) may be more difficult to exclude. Leiomyomas are again primarily intramural lesions. Also, they are generally not quite as soft as the lipomas. Mostly, they appear as reasonably firm, round masses, frequently with central ulcerations. Nevertheless, it has to be kept in mind that some leiomyomas are very fleshy and very flexible. An adenomatous polyp (D) would be one of the hardest differential diagnoses. The striking roundness and the very obvious radiolucency are in favor of lipoma although thes features are difficult to evaluate quantitatively in the average examination.

QUESTION 104

Of the offered choices, (C) copious mucous secretions is the most correct. The villous adenoma contains large amounts of mucus-produc-ing glands and cells. Vigorous production of mucus, therefore, is charac-teristic and may be serious enough to bring the patient into electrolyte imbalance. (A) is not correct. Villous adenoma is ordinarily a solitary le-sion. Marked radiolucency (B) is typical of lipoma. All the other polypoid lesions of the colon, including villous adenoma, adenoma, polypoid carcinoma, and hamartoma, are of "water density." A smooth surface (D) is obviously an incorrect answer in view of the frond-covered surface of the usual villous adenoma. The "common location" of the villous adenoma in the small intestine is incorrect (E). The colon is the most common organ for villous adenoma, especially in the rectum and the sigmoid.

QUESTION 105

The correct answer is (D)—intestinal endometriosis generally *is* **associated with symptoms.** The lesion frequently will contain fluid which may be the result of degenerated blood products. There may be cyclic bleeding into the lesion during menstrual periods. The lesion furthermore may bleed into the intestinal lumen, frequently in a cyclic fashion, but not necessarily so. Also, it sets up considerable local irritation and may lead to inflammatory and fibrotic changes. The other answers are correct statements about endometriosis and, therefore, not the right answers to this question. Obstruction may be produced by the fibrotic contraction caused by the reaction to the endometriosis. Occasionally, the mass may be large enough to compress the bowel. Due to the location of the sigmoid colon (next to the gynecological organs), that portion of the colon indeed is the most common location of endometriosis. Endometriosis primarily is a lesion of gynecological organs but the implantation on the intestinal tract is not unusual. The lesions frequently are multiple and may be of varying sizes. The most common radiological manifestation is an intramural mass associated with what appears to be a roundish pressure deformity and some element of constriction of the bowel at the site of the lesion.

QUESTION 106

The most common location of lipoma is the colon (E). Of the other choices, the small bowel (C) is probably the next most common. In the duodenum, a soft, smooth, approximately 1-cm. lesion is likely to be a lipoma. In the esophagus (A) and jejunum, they are quite unusual. In the stomach (B) and the ileum (D), they are a bit more common. In the colon, the most common location is the cecum and ascending colon.

DISCUSSION

Lipomas most commonly occur in patients past middle age. The lesions are invariably benign and appear as intramural lesions. They are generally about 1 to 3 cm. in diameter. About one third are pedunculated. Because of their pedunculated nature, intussusception may be a complication and in some series has occurred in up to 40 per cent of the cases. Traction on

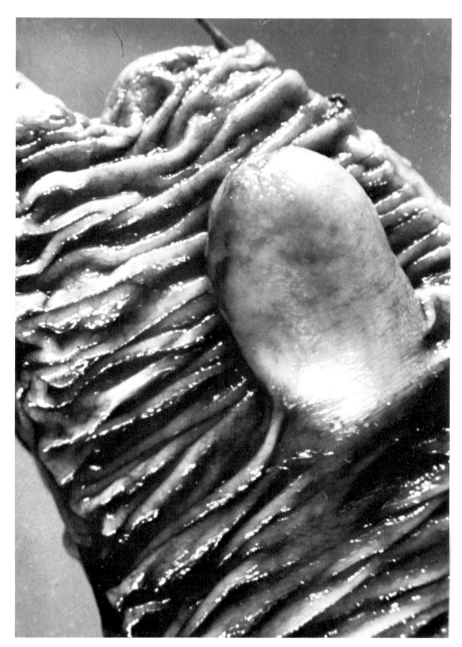

Figure 52A

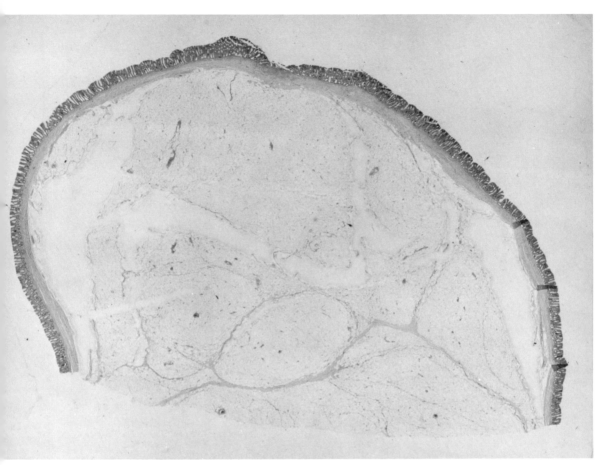

Figure 52B

the polyp by peristalsis or intermittent intussusceptions may account for the attacks of crampy pain that some of the patients have. In about one third of the cases, the lipoma is an incidental finding in asymptomatic patients or in patients being examined for other reasons. Ulceration occurs occasionally. Figure 52A is a photograph of the resected lesion in this case. Figure 52B is a low power enlargement. Note the very "empty" fatty interior structures of a typical lipoma and the normal, uninterrupted, smooth mucosa covering the lesion.

Differentiation of a lipoma from a carcinoma is not difficult since the lipoma is not circumferential and generally is quite smooth. Differentiation from a benign adenomatous polyp may be more difficult because the latter can also be quite smooth. The roentgen findings as seen in the classical case include relative radiolucency of the lesion (especially as compared to surrounding soft tissue density in an area immediately adjacent to the involved portion of the colon), softness of the lesion (best demonstrated by showing a change in shape or apparent size on compression), and a strikingly smooth surface. Water enemas have been recommended as a possible tool of differential diagnosis, since a lipoma, due to its fat content, will be more radiolucent than the surrounding water. An interesting side-light is the occasional spontaneous expulsion of intestinal lipomas, apparently by the mechanism of intussusception with subsequent necrosis of the stalk. The lesion may be so soft that it may be missed on palpation of the bowel from the outside during surgical exploration.

The softness of the lesion frequently produces the "squeeze" sign cf lipoma (on postevacuation films the lesion which on filled films appears rounded, becomes oblong and sausage-shaped).

Another entity to be mentioned is lipomatosis of the ileocecal valve, a totally benign and most likely not even neoplastic lesion. The fatty infiltration is diffuse. In these cases, the ileocecal valve appears unusually prominent and quite smooth. Increased radiolucency generally cannot be identified. The main lesion in differential diagnosis is carcinoma. The smoothness and the regular appearance are the prime diagnostic criteria in favor of lipomatosis.

SUGGESTED READINGS

1. Castro EB, Stearns MW: Lipoma of the large intestine. A review of 45 cases. Dis Colon & Rectum 15:441–444, 1972
2. Margulis AR, Jovanovich A: The roentgen diagnosis of submucous lipomas of the colon. Am J Roentgenol 84:1114–1120, 1960
3. Palazzo WL: Lipomas of the gastrointestinal tract. Am J Roentgenol 62:825–830, 1949
4. Seaman WB: Disease of the colon. New concepts, old problems. Radiology 100:251–269, 1971
5. Wolf BS: Roentgen features of benign tumors of the colon. Surg Clin North Am 45:1141–1155, 1965
6. Stevens GM: The use of a water enema in the verification of lipoma of the colon. Am J Roentgenol 96:292–297, 1966

CORRECT ANSWERS

Question 103-(E)
Question 104-(C)
Question 105-(D)
Question 106-(E)

NOTES

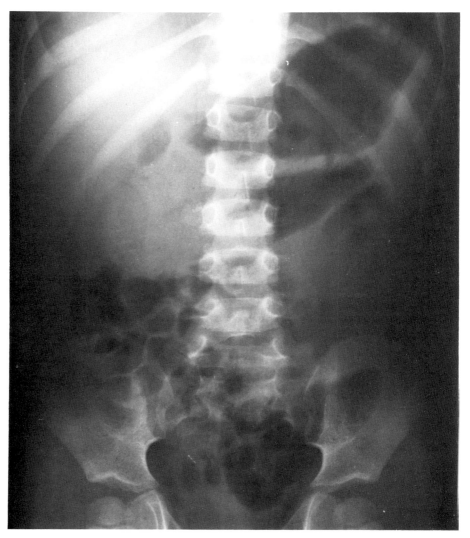

Figure 53. This 3-year-old boy has severe, intermittent abdominal pain of 3 hours' duration. Your are shown a plain roentgenogram of the abdomen taken with the patient in the supine position.

Questions 107 through 109

107. Which one of the following is the *MOST* likely diagnosis?

   (A)   Renal abscess
   (B)   Ileocolic intussusception
   (C)   Gastric outlet obstruction
   (D)   "Closed loop" obstruction
   (E)   Suprarenal hematoma

108. Which one of the following is *LEAST* likely to be associated with a soft tissue mass seen on plain roentgenograms of the abdomen?

   (A)   Hydronephrosis
   (B)   Intussusception
   (C)   Appendicitis
   (D)   Hypertrophic pyloric stenosis
   (E)   Choledochal cyst

109. Which one of the following statements concerning the use of enemas in ileocolic intussusception in young children is *CORRECT*?

   (A)   A carefully performed barium enema is effective and accepted treatment in many cases
   (B)   It should not be used as treatment for intussusception
   (C)   A barium enema can be used to reduce the intussusception, but this should always be followed by surgical exploration
   (D)   If the intussusception cannot be reduced easily, the barium enema fluid pressure should be increased
   (E)   Postevacuation films are of little use

Discussion

QUESTION 107

Ileocolic intussusception (B) is the diagnosis in this case. A rounded soft tissue mass (Figure 53A, "A" arrows), about 5 cm. in diameter, is seen between the air in the duodenal bulb (Figure 53A, "B" arrow) and the lower ileal loops (Figure 53A, "C" arrows). There is *more* than an average amount of gas in the lower ileum and *less* than an average amount of gas in the colon. The combination of these two findings suggests a low small bowel obstruction. In the presence of a soft tissue mass in the right upper quadrant, in this age group, a small bowel obstruction due to intussusception is most likely.

A barium enema was performed on this patient. Figure 53B shows barium filling the transverse colon from the direction of the splenic flexure (spot roentgenogram 1). A typical, rounded intraluminal mass is outlined by the advancing barium which extends slightly along the upper edge of the mass. Spot roentgenogram 2 (Figure 53B) shows increasing mild distention of the transverse colon as the infusion of barium suspension continues. The intussuscepted mass has receded to the hepatic flexure. On spot roentgenogram 3 (Figure 53B) the mass is now located in the upper descending colon. Lastly, spot roentgenogram 4 (Figure 53B) shows a normally filled cecum with barium passing retrograde through the ileocecal valve filling the terminal ileum. The intussusception has been reduced by the barium enema.

A renal abscess (A) is less likely because the mass appears smaller than the kidney would be expected to be, especially in vertical diameter. Also there are no gas bubbles in the lesion (although not all renal abscesses contain gas bubbles), and in addition the intestinal gas distribution here makes an extraintestinal lesion less likely than one within the intestinal tract itself. Gastric outlet obstruction (C) is not very likely because the stomach is not dilated and does not show the deep incisive peristaltic waves seen with pyloric obstruction in small children. Also, a fair amount of gas is present in the intestinal tract beyond the pylorus. In pyloric stenosis, however, gas is often present in normal amounts in the more distal portions of the intestinal tract. "Closed loop" obstruction (D) is also much less likely since the so-called "coffee bean", double-lumen appearance is not seen here. While much fluid accumulates frequently in the dilated loops, in closed loop obstructions there often also is a small amount of air helping to identify the loop (see Figure 20B, p. 111). While it would be conceivable that the soft tissue mass seen in the right upper abdomen in this case could be such a fluid-filled, twisted loop, closed loop obstructions in this age group most commonly involve volvulus of the midgut, which would involve a much larger part of the intestinal tract. A single loop in the right upper quadrant would indeed be an unusual site of volvulus in a small child. A suprarenal hematoma (E) would be expected to be higher in the abdomen on the right side, or, if it were displacing the kidney downward, to result in a lower kidney shadow. If such a retroperitoneal hematoma were no larger than the mass found in this case, it would unlikely cause as much displacement of small bowel and right colon gas as is evident here. In small children retroperitoneal masses can displace intestinal gas more readily than in adults. However, such masses need to be of considerable size so as to protrude from the retroperitoneal area into the peritoneal cavity, taking up space ordinarily occupied by intestinal structures.

QUESTION 108

All of the listed diseases may be associated with soft tissue mases. In the case of hydronephrosis (A), the mass is caused by the dilated renal pelvis and collecting system causing an enlarged kidney; in intussusception (B) by the intussuscepted intestinal mass; in appendicitis (C) by the periappendiceal cellulitis or frequently the appendiceal abscess; and lastly, in choledochal cyst (E), by the cyst itself. However, **hypertrophic pyloric stenosis ((D) the correct answer for this question)** is *not* associated with a mass visible on plain roentgenograms of the abdomen. The hypertrophic pyloric muscle mass in these infants is frequently palpable in the upper abdomen, especially if good relaxation of the patient's abdominal musculature can be achieved. Nevertheless, the mass is usually small enough and surrounded by other water-density structures so that it is not apparent on plain films. This results in the somewhat paradoxical situation that the small mass of pyloric hypertrophy may be more readily palpable on careful examination), and yet is less obvious radiologically.

QUESTION 109

The correct answer is (A). In many cases the intussusception can be reduced readily by barium enema. Besides avoiding a needless surgical procedure in many cases, earlier reduction may prevent necrosis of the intussuscepted bowel by earlier elimination or decrease of ischemia. Most intussusceptions in young children are not associated with a leading mass; therefore, if the intussusception can be reduced and remains reduced, surgical intervention is unnecessary. The situation is different in adults where intussusception most commonly is caused by a neoplastic mass. There, even though the intussusception may be reduced by barium enema, surgical treatment is still necessary to eliminate the underlying lesion.

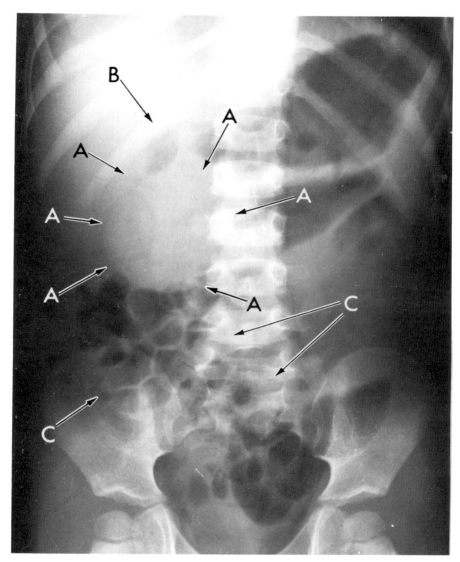

Figure 53A

(B) is incorrect in view of what was just said. The contraindications to barium-enema reduction of intussusception include the danger of perforation if *peritonitis* or *extreme clinical conditions* are present or the intussusception has persisted for a long time. As a general rule, in both children and adults, *any* type of enema is undesirable if a perforation of the colon is suspected. This applies to barium enemas, Gastrografin enemas, saline and water enemas. Any enema under these circumstances may wash bacterially contaminated fecal material from the colon into the peritoneal cavity and aggravate the situation. There is some evidence that the presence of barium sulfate particles may make the resulting peritonitis worse by virtue of the presence of nonresorbable foreign material. (C) is incorrect because if the intussusception is reduced and remains reduced in small children, follow-up surgery is unnecessary. It is, however, necessary to take a careful look at a postevacuation film because occasionally the intussusception will recur during the evacuation of the barium suspension.

If the intussusception cannot be reduced easily with a barium enema, the barium enema fluid pressure should *not* be increased (D). Please see the discussion of barium enema reduction in the discussion section below. Postevacuation films (E) should be obtained and are important because of the possibility of recurrent intussusception.

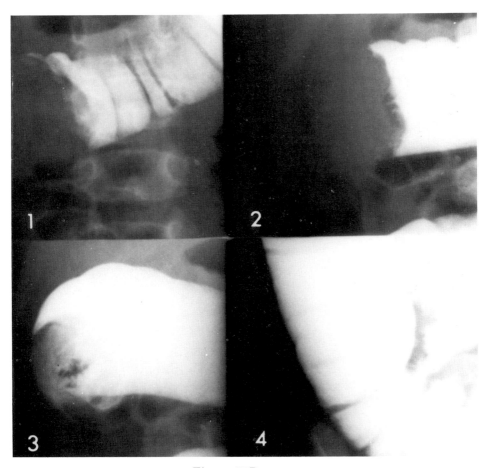

Figure 53B

DISCUSSION (also see discussion on pp. 232–237)

Intussusception is the invagination of a portion of the intestinal tract into the intestinal lumen and then downward propulsion of the resulting "mass" by peristaltic activity. Once a lead point of this type has been established, there is gradual progression of this structure downward, pulling behind it more and more of the intestine which now "telescopes" into itself. This leads to a varying but usually considerable degree of obstruction which eventually becomes complete. Also, if the process continues for some time, the vascular supply is compromised and the ischemic intussuscepted bowel undergoes necrosis. Intussusception in adults usually is the result of some type of a leading lesion (a mass, which often is either polypoid or one that is not fixed by invasion through the wall; less commonly, enlarged lymphoid patches in the wall of the bowel or a Meckel's diverticulum may serve this purpose). Small bowel intussusceptions limited to the small bowel may occur on an intermittent basis and self reduce. These need to be considered in the differential diagnosis in patients who complain of attacks of crampy abdominal pain, especially after eating. Even in the infant with ileocolic intussusception the severity may vary and the symptoms and signs may fluctuate.

The main area of interest in this discussion is the most common type of intussusception, the *ileocolic intussusception* in the small child. This is a characteristic entity occurring most commonly in infants under 2 years of age, and usually over the age of 3 months. There is a predominance in male infants. The onset is fairly rapid with intermittent abdominal pain, which may be very severe. A mass is often palpable, most commonly in the right side of the abdomen, either in the lower portion or in the right upper quadrant. It may change location and, if located in the cecal area, may be most readily discovered by bimanual rectal and abdominal examination. Blood in the stool is very commonly present and is said to be of "current jelly" appearance frequently.

If diagnosis is made early, the prognosis is quite good. Mortality is under 1 per cent among infants who are relieved of the condition within 24 hours. After 48 hours, the mortality increases very rapidly. It seems that without treatment almost all children would die. The number of spontaneous reductions is unknown. It is to be noted that of the purely small bowel intussusception in adults (jejunojejunal, jejunoileal, or ileoileal), a fair number intermittently self reduce and opinions have been expressed that the so-called "colic" of the very small infant may be due to temporary ileoileal intussusceptions. Self reduction of ileocolic intussusception is considered possible, but waiting for this spontaneous event of unknown frequency is hazardous. If intussusception is suspected, the lesion should be treated. Expectant observation is not acceptable in view of the high incidence of necrosis and mortality in untreated cases. Once the diagnosis is suspected clinically, roentgenograms will almost invariably be obtained. In early cases (it is desirable to establish the diagnosis early) there may be no evidence of small bowel obstruction. If there is clinical suspicion of intussusception, one should proceed with the barium enema. Nevertheless, it is often possible to identify vaguely a soft tissue mass somewhere in the right abdomen and some discrepancy in gas distribution, as is evident in this case.

The barium enema is performed in much the same way as any barium enema would be done in a small infant. The container for the barium enema should be between 24 and 36 inches above the level of the anus of the patient. An unlubricated, not too small (slow flow!) soft rubber catheter is inserted in the anus and the buttocks then taped together with adhesive tape, passing the tape around the catheter to prevent removal by slight accidental traction. Some radiologists advocate the use of a balloon-type catheter. This is acceptable, but one should make quite sure that it is not *excessively inflated*. The balloon should be inflated with a large syringe after a small amount of barium outlines the rectum. The balloon, when inflated, should rest against the walls of the rectum *and no more*. Overinflation of retention balloons in the rectum of infants is one of the commonest causes of iatrogenic perforation of the rectum, a clinical disaster. One should proceed gradually and avoid manual pressure on the abdomen. The reduction of the intussusception by the enema may occur rapidly or may proceed gradually over a period of 10 minutes or so. If reduction does not occur easily, one should not engage in a prolonged attempt. If only partial reduction can be achieved, something of value has been accomplished since it will make surgical reduction easier and may delay ischemic necrosis of the intussusception. Re-reduction of recurrent intussusception is acceptable. If recurrences reoccur after such attempts, surgical treatment becomes necessary. One should make sure that the intussusception is reduced completely. Frye and Howard (see suggested readings list) have described one such technique used successfully at an active pediatric hospital.

The diagnostic findings on the barium enema during the reduction procedure include the presence of a convex intracolonic mass outlined by barium and an apparent obstruction to retrograde flow of barium. Fairly frequently one will see the barium extending around the periphery of the intussuscepted mass. The mucosal pattern then produces the characteristic "coil spring" appearance. Occasionally one will see some suggestion of an internal lumen of the intussuscepted bowel filling with barium.

This, however, is more common in the small bowel intussusceptions when barium is given by mouth (see Figure 50B, p. 234). If the intussusception is completely reduced, or partially reduced, and recurs, the postevacuation film will show the rather characteristic "coil spring" appearance with barium around the intussuscepted segment of bowel.

A surgeon should be notified as soon as the diagnosis is suspected because an operation may be necessary. Occasionally, the residual edema or lymphocytic hyperplasia of the ileocecal valve may cause some difficulty on postevacuation films by simulating persistent intussusception.

SUGGESTED READINGS

1. Caffey J: *Pediatric X-ray Diagnosis*, 6th ed, pp 661–666. Year Book Medica. Publishers, Chicago, 1972
2. Frye TR, Howard WHF: Handling of ileocolic intussusception in pediatric medical centers (editorial). Radiology 97:187–191, 1970.
3. Ling J: Intussusception in infants and children with emphasis on the recognition of cases with complications. Radiology 62:505–513, 1954
4. Middlemiss JH: Intussusception in childhood: radiologic appearance in plain radiographs. Brit J Radiol 28:257–263, 1955
5. Ravitch MM: *Intussusception in Infants and Children*. Charles C Thomas, Springfield, Ill, 1959

CORRECT ANSWERS

Question 107-(B)
Question 108-(D)
Question 109-(A)

NOTES

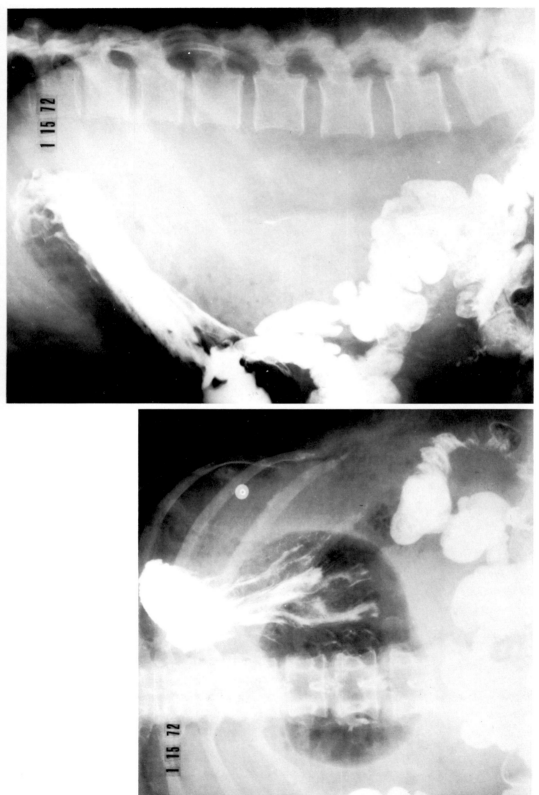

Figures 54 (left) and 55 (right). This 41-year-old woman has acute abdominal pain and fever. You are shown anteroposterior (Figure 54) and lateral (Figure 55) views of an upper GI series.

Questions 110 and 111

110. Which one of the following is the *MOST* likely diagnosis?

   (A)   Carcinoma of the pancreas
   (B)   Pseudocyst of the pancreas
   (C)   Emphysematous gastritis
   (D)   Abscess of the lesser sac
   (E)   Perforated duodenal ulcer

111. A decrease in serum calcium level in a patient with an "acute abdomen" should *MOST* likely suggest which one of the following diagnoses?

   (A)   Small bowel obstruction
   (B)   Acute pancreatitis
   (C)   Pseudocyst of the pancreas
   (D)   Acute pyelonephritis
   (E)   Perforated hollow viscus

Discussion

QUESTION 110

Figures 54 and 55 show numerous gas bubbles behind the anteriorly displaced stomach extending both to the right and left of the spine. **The most likely diagnosis with this roentgen finding is an abscess of the lesser sac (D).**

Although carcinoma or pseudocyst of the pancreas could cause such displacement, the gas bubbles essentially exclude these diagnoses.

Emphysematous gastritis is an unusual variant of phlegmonous gastritis due to invasion of the gastric wall by gas-forming organisms. Onset of the disease is explosive and the course fulminating, with a high mortality rate. Generally the condition follows a pre-existing gastrointestinal illness, operation, or after ingestion of caustics. The roentgen findings of emphysematous gastritis are characteristic in that the gas bubbles outline the stomach (Figure 55A, along greater curvature), as opposed to an abscess of the lesser sac. Barium studies are of further help in demonstrating gas bubbles in the gastric wall. In addition, dissection of barium into the wall is often seen (Figure 55B, along greater curvature).

Although perforated duodenal ulcer can result in a lesser sac abscess if the perforation is posterior, there are multiple causes of lesser sac abscess and, therefore, this answer is not as good as (D), abscess of the lesser sac.

The majority of lesser sac abscesses are related to pancreatitis. Other causes include posterior perforation of the stomach, extension of liver abscesses, cholecystitis, and leakage of retrocolic gastrojejunostomy. Therefore, any inflammatory process in the *vicinity* of the lesser sac can result in the formation of such an abscess. In almost all patients there is notable displacement of the stomach and duodenum or other neighboring viscera. Generally speaking, the stomach is displaced anteriorly but occasionally it may actually be displaced posteriorly due to anterior extension of the abscess into the lesser omentum or the gastrocolic ligament.

The recognition of a lesser sac abscess is not difficult if the cavity is large and contains a fluid level. However, in the absence of a fluid level, gas in the upper part of the lesser sac may simulate pneumoperitoneum on erect films. Generally speaking, however, the abscesses are manifested as in this case by multiple tiny gas bubbles which remain unchanged in position.

QUESTION 111

The answer to question 111 is acute pancreatitis (B). The hallmark of acute pancreatitis is peritoneal fat necrosis which is almost specific for this disease. In addition to the abdomen it may also be seen in other areas of the body including bone marrow, subcutaneous tissue, muscle, liver, bladder, lungs, heart, and renal capsule. In the presence of pancreatitis, neutral fat undergoes hydrolysis to glycerol and fatty acid, the glycerol being absorbed and the fatty acid being precipitated with calcium. This nodule of fat necrosis is actually a deposition of calcium soaps. Alteration in calcium metabolism is related to this deposition of the calcium soap. In pancreatitis the amount of calcium deposited in the pancreas and surrounding tissues may easily equal or exceed the total normal circulating calcium; therefore, a marked fall in the serum calcium is seen and tetany may be present.

Unlike most radiographic findings in acute pancreatitis, the roentgen manifestation of peritoneal fat necrosis is specific. The findings are *rare*, however, and require good quality films to be seen. The pattern consists of mottled lucencies representing normal fat, interspersed with areas of water density representing the hydrolization products (Figure 55C, *arrows*).

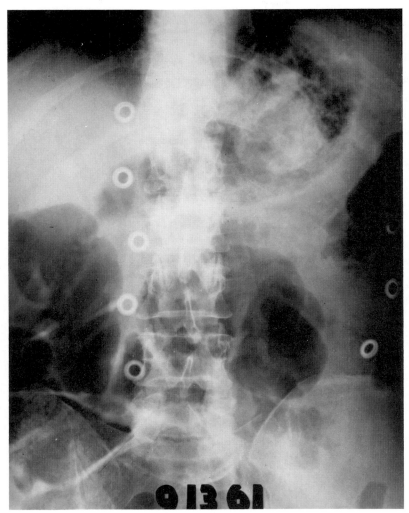

Figure 55A

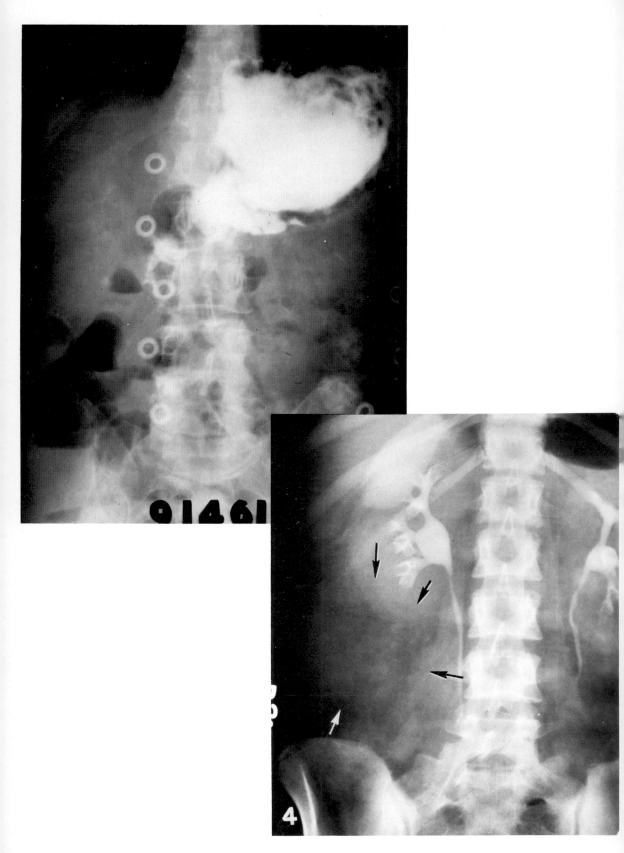

Figures 55B (top) and C (bottom)

Although most prominent in the area of the pancreas they may extend for considerable distance from it and when seen are a poor prognostic sign.

None of the other suggested entities in question 111 can cause significant decrease in serum calcium levels in themselves.

SUGGESTED READINGS

1. Berenson JE, Spitz HB, Felson B: The abdominal fat necrosis sign. Radiology *100:*567–571, 1971
2. Felson B: Gas abscess of pancreas. JAMA *163:*637–641, 1957
3. Gonzalez LL, Schowengerdt C, Skinner HH Jr, Lynch P: Emphysematous gastritis. Surg Gynecol & Obstet *116:*79–87, 1963
4. Howard JM: Physiologic changes associated with acute pancreatitis. In JM Howard, GL Jordan Jr (eds): *Surgical Diseases of the Pancreas*, pp 116–122. JB Lippincott Co, Philadelphia, 1960
5. Mellins HZ: The radiologic signs of disease in the lesser peritoneal sac. Radiol Clin North Am *2:*107–120, 1964
6. Nelson SW: Extraluminal gas collections due to diseases of the gastrointestinal tract. Am J Roentgenol *115:*225–248, 1972
7. Walker LA, Weens HS: Radiological observations on the lesser peritoneal sac. Radiology *80:*727–737, 1963

CORRECT ANSWERS

Question 110-(D)
Question 111-(B)

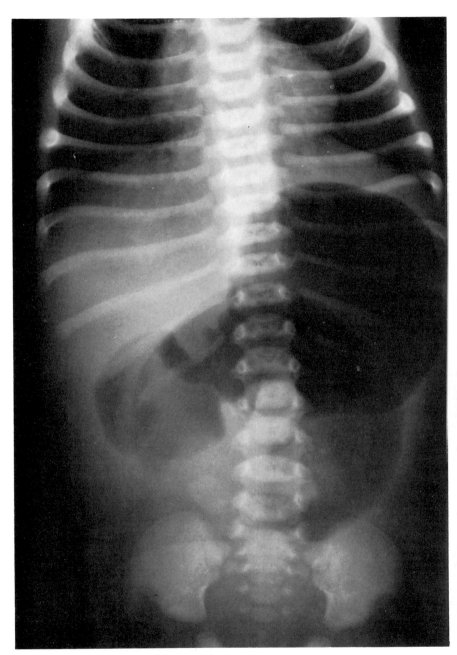

Figure 56

Figures 56 and 57. This 3-day-old girl is vomiting and has abdominal distension. Roentgenograms were taken with the patient in the supine (Figure 56) and upright (Figure 57) positions.

Questions 112 through 117

112. Which one of the following is the *MOST* likely diagnosis?

    (A)   Congenital antral diaphragm
    (B)   Hypertrophic pyloric stenosis
    (C)   Annular pancreas
    (D)   Jejunal atresia
    (E)   Ileal atresia

For each of the numbered clinical disorders listed below (Questions 113–117), select the *one* lettered clinical roentgenographic manifestation (A,B,C,D,E) that is *MOST* closely associated with it. Each lettered clinical roentgenographic manifestation may be selected once, more than once, or not at all.

    (A)   Frequently diagnosed by clinical manifestations alone
    (B)   Decreased iliac index
    (C)   Obstructing peritoneal band
    (D)   Severe microcolon
    (E)   Obstruction relieved by Gastrografin or other enema

113. Duodenal atresia

114. Midgut malrotation

115. "Meconium plug" syndrome

116. Ileal atresia

117. Hypertrophic pyloric stenosis

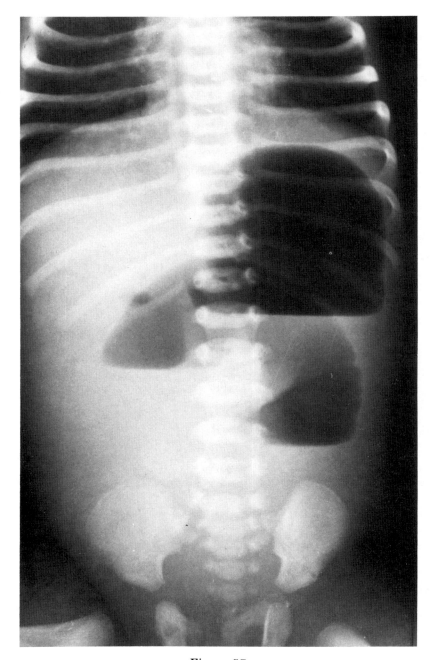

Figure 57

Discussion

QUESTION 112

Jejunal atresia (D) is the correct answer. Air is seen in the stomach, the duodenum, and one large jejunal loop ("C" *arrows*, Figures 57A and B). The more distal loops contain no air at all. While there is marked distention of the stomach with gas and while there is a large gas-containing loop in the mid abdomen, this is *not* the "double bubble" sign of annular pancreas (C) or duodenal atresia. The presence of a dilated gas-containing organ distal to the stomach excludes congenital antral diaphragm (A) and hypertrophic pyloric stenosis (B), both of which produce gastric outlet obstruction. While gas is often present in the intestinal tract in normal amounts in both conditions, distention of more distal bowel loops does not occur unless there is another lesion. Ileal atresia (E) is probably the most difficult differential diagnosis to exclude. Not infrequently, with low small bowel obstructions, the lowermost portion of the distended small bowel is totally filled with fluid, does not contain air in perceptible amounts, and, therefore, is not readily identified on roentgenograms. Therefore, a *low* small bowel obstruction may at times simulate a *high* bowel obstruction. In this case, however, there is only *one* markedly distended small bowel loop in the mid abdomen. Usually, with low small bowel obstruction there are at least two or three dilated upper small bowel loops with gas in them. Air is seen in the second portion of the duodenum ("*A*" *arrows*, Figure 57A) and a small air bubble rises into the duodenal bulb on the upright view (Figure 57A, "*B*" *arrow*). If this bubble were much larger and if the curved mid abdominal gas-containing loop were not seen, the possibility of annular pancreas or duodenal atresia might have been entertained.

The following are matched numbered clinical disorders and lettered clinical roentgenographic manifestations:

QUESTION 113

Duodenal atresia occurs with increased frequency in patients with Down's syndrome (mongolism). The **iliac index (B),** as described by Caffey and Ross, is one of the roentgenographic signs of the Down's syndrome. In mongoloid newborn infants the acetabular and iliac angles are *smaller* than normal.

QUESTION 114

Midgut malrotation may lead to a midgut volvulus. However, in many cases an acute volvulus does not develop; rather, **peritoneal bands (C),**

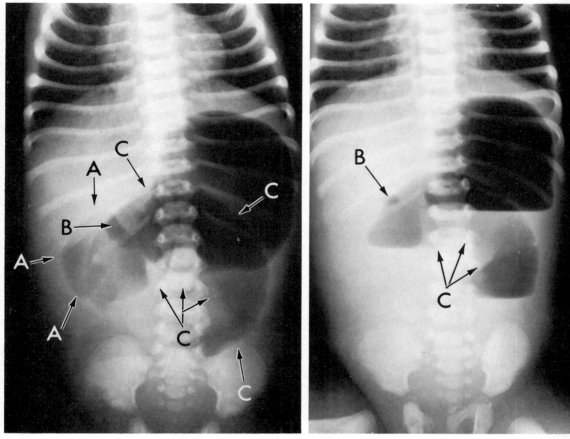

Figure 57A   Figure 57B

sometimes called Ladd's bands, extend in various directions. A very common location of these bands is across the lower portion of the duodenal sweep (in the area of the third part of the duodenum). These bands cause episodes of acute obstruction, or more commonly, episodes of partial obstruction. These may be aggravated by food intake with increase of symptoms after eating, and in certain positions (standing may cause tightening of the bands and increase in symptoms while lying down may relax them). Barium studies of the gastrointestinal tract may show evidence of near complete or partial obstruction of the duodenum at this point. In many cases, however, not much evidence of obstruction is seen and the diagnosis has to be made on the basis of the presence of malrotation as identified on the barium enema or upper gastrointestinal studies (see Figures 17D through G, p. 99).

In an acute midgut volvulus these bands may produce a complete obstruction of the duodenum, resulting in a "double bubble" sign, otherwise typical of duodenal atresia or annular pancreas (one "bubble" is air in the dilated stomach, the other is air in the proximal part of the duodenum) (see Figures 16 and 17, pp 92 and 94).

QUESTION 115

The "meconium plug" syndrome is associated with **relief of obstruction by enemas (E).** In fact, this entity, which consists simply of a local inspissation of meconium leading to a low colon obstruction, frequently is relieved spontaneously by normal expulsion of meconium and occasionally by rectal examination or the insertion of a thermometer. Sometimes these plugs are more persistent than average. Enemas, therefore, may dislodge them and return the patient to normal. Gastrografin has been described as being particularly effective, apparently due to its hypertonic nature and stimulation of peristalsis. The entity is a common one and ordinarily relieved quite easily.

Frech *et al.* and Noblett have even described this method in the treatment of *meconium ileus* (a disease in which the meconium is abnormal due to mucoviscidosis) in contrast to the *meconium plug* (which is understood to occur with otherwise normal meconium). The danger of hypertonicity has to be kept in mind when using a Gastrografin enema (Rowe *et al.*) and the infants should be followed closely with appropriate tests and their fluid and electrolyte balance maintained.

QUESTION 116

In ileal atresia little or no small bowel contents (which in the fetus consist of desquamated cells, bile, the products of intestinal secretion, etc.) reach the colon. The presence of such material in the colon in the normal fetus results in a mild increase in the size of the colon producing what we recognize as a *normal* infantile colon. In the absence of such material, the colon remains quite thin and ribbon-like. This is known as a **microcolon (D)** and is most characteristically seen with complete low small bowel obstructions. The higher the obstruction in the intestinal tract, the less pronounced is the microcolon. With duodenal atresias the appearance of the colon may be similar to that seen in normal infants. Incidentally, some of this effect is also noted in adults in that patients who have had colostomies to divert the fecal stream for a long time will show decrease in the size of the more distal portion of the colon.

It is of some importance to note that barium enemas in small infants should generally be performed by using isotonic saline or a similar solution as a medium for suspension of the barium since, in those cases where the enema may be retained (such as in Hirschsprung's disease), *water intoxication* may develop and may be fatal. *Hypertonic fluids* tend to attract water into the colon and, hence, if Gastrografin or other hypertonic materials are used, the possibility of *dehydration* of the patient should be watched for.

QUESTION 117

Hypertonic pyloric stenosis is frequently diagnosed by clinical manifestations alone (A). The disease develops characteristically in male infants a few weeks after birth, is associated with projectile vomiting and, with care (especially making sure that the abdominal wall is relaxed) an olive-shaped small mass can be palpated in the area of the pylorus. These findings may be sufficient to establish the diagnosis and lead to surgical treatment. Roentgen examination, however, is ordinarily used to confirm the diagnosis and help clarify obscure cases. It shows the characteristic findings of elongation and narrowing of the pyloric canal, frequently with a slight bend, as well as a mass impression upon the distal-most part of the antrum of the stomach and the proximal surface of the duodenal bulb. Signs of gastric obstruction, dilatation and active hyperperistalsis, are usually evident.

DISCUSSION

Atresia of the small bowel is a congenital defect whose cause is not determined. One popular opinion has been that it is due to a lack of recanalization of the lumen of that part of the intestinal tract in the course of development. Recently, other causes have been proposed, including suggestions that atresia may be a lesion acquired *in utero* caused by local ischemia, volvulus, intussusception, and other mechanisms leading to local necrosis and "incorrect" healing. Experimental obstruction of mesenteric blood vessels in developing animals has produced similar lesions.

Wolfson and Williams have alerted us to the fact that some of these infants with small bowel atresia have direct, open communication of the small intestinal lumen *distal* to the atresia with the peritoneal cavity. They recommend special care in performing enemas on patients with such atresias.

Intrauterine perforations of the intestine in patients with small bowel atresia may lead to meconium peritonitis, a condition which may be identified by virtue of calcifications in the peritoneal cavity seen on roentgenograms. These perforations are frequently not found to be open at the time of surgery. This process may be secondary support for the theory of ischemia as a cause for the atresia, as may be the presence of the occasional persistent perforations downstream from the atresia described by Wolfson and Williams.

Aside from the peritoneal calcifications associated with meconium peritonitis (seen in only some cases of atresia) the manifestations of these atresias in the newborn are much the same as those of any small bowel obstruction. One looks for the dilated small intestinal loops with fluid levels. A few points of special interest need to be remembered in the pediatric age group as compared to adults. It is difficult, and frequently impossible, to clearly separate the appearance of the colon from that of the small bowel in infants less than 2 years old. Thus, the plain film differentiation between a *colon* obstruction and a *small bowel* obstruction in infants may be impossible and cannot be relied upon. Barium studies, preferably beginning with a barium enema, are required to make this differentiation. Meconium ileus, a lesion of infants resulting from defective excretion of enzymes into the intestinal tract in patients with cystic fibrosis of the pancreas, causes an appearance similar to that of a small bowel obstruction. However, in many cases, the fluid levels are not as clearly evident as they are in the simple mechanical small bowel obstructions and, in fact, the unusually viscid intestinal contents on the roentgen films appear bubbly and irregularly distributed.

Midgut volvulus is another cause for acute small bowel obstruction in the newborn infant or shortly after birth. Three basic patterns are found in midgut volvulus: (1) a *high* small bowel obstruction with gas in the stomach and the duodenum (suggesting the "double bubble" sign) or one additional jejunal loop and a lack of gas more distally; (2) a *low* bowel obstruction with multiple dilated midabdominal small bowel loops with fluid levels; and (3) normal abdomen, which, when coupled with bile-containing vomitus, should suggest the possibility of the diagnosis and is an indication of further roentgen studies (barium enema or upper gastrointestinal examination).

In the study of small bowel obstructions in the pediatric age group, the barium enema is a very crucial method of examination and ordinarily should be the next step after the plain films. In the case of malrotation with duodenal bands and in midgut volvulus, the abnormal colon position identifies the developmental abnormality and permits one to make the diagnosis. Intussusception is another common cause for intestinal obstruction in the pediatric age group. Again, the most common type of intussusception is the ileocolic, and the barium enema is the cornerstone of diagnosis. The presence or absence of a microcolon and the identification of the meconium plug help identify the intestinal atresias and the meconium plug syndrome. The characteristic changes in the diameter of the colon, sometimes the fold pattern in the rectum, and the prolonged retention of barium in the colon identify Hirschsprung's disease or congenital megacolon.

Some radiologists prefer to administer barium by mouth first. We believe that the ability to spontaneously evacuate barium from the colon in small infants and the information obtained suggests advantages in doing a barium enema first.

Treatment of atresia obviously is surgical. It is important to make the diagnosis promptly because small bowel obstruction is associated with a high mortality, even in the adult, but especially in the pediatric age group.

SUGGESTED READINGS

SMALL BOWEL ATRESIA

1. Grosfeld JL, Clatworthy HW Jr: The nature of ileal atresia due to intrauterine intussusception. Arch Surg 100:714–717, 1970
2. Nixon HH, Tawes R: Etiology and treatment of small intestinal atresia: analysis of a series of 127 jejunoileal atresias and comparison with 62 duodenal atresias. Surgery 69:41–51, 1971
3. Wolfson, JJ, Williams H: Hazard of barium enema studies in infants with small bowel atresia. Radiology 95: 341–343, 1970

MIDGUT VOLVULUS

1. Berdon WE, Baker DH, Bull S, Santulli TV: Midgut malrotation and volvulus. Which films are best? Radiology 96: 375–383, 1970
2. Frye TR, Mah CL, Schiller M: Roentgenographic evidence of gangrenous bowel in midgut volvulus with observations in experimental volvulus. Am J Roentgenol 114: 394–401, 1972
3. Pochaczevsky R, Ratner H, Leonidas JC, Naysan P, Ferraru F: Unusual forms of volvulus after the neonatal period. Am J Roentgenol 114: 390–393, 1972

PELVIC INDEX IN DOWN'S SYNDROME

Caffey J, Ross S: Pelvic bones in infantile mongoloidism: radiographic features. Am J Roentgenol 80: 458–467, 1958

MECONIUM PLUG SYNDROME AND HYPERTONIC ENEMAS

1. Frech RS, McAlister WH, Ternberg J, Strominger, D: Meconium ileus relieved by 40% water-soluble contrast enemas. Radiology 94: 341–342, 1970
2. Noblett HR: Treatment of uncomplicated meconium ileus by Gastrografin enemas: a preliminary report. Pediat Surg 4: 190–197, 1959
3. Rowe MI, Seagram G, Weinberger M: Gastrografin-induced hypertonicity. The pathogenesis of a neonatal hazard. Am J Surg 125: 185–188, 1973
4. Roe MI, Furst AJ, Altman DH, Poole CA: Neonatal response to Gastrografin enemas. Pediatrics 48: 29–35, 1971

CORRECT ANSWERS

Question 112-(D)
Question 113-(B)
Question 114-(C)
Question 115-(E)
Question 116-(D)
Question 117-(A)

NOTES

Table of Contents

The Table of Contents is placed in this unusual location so that the reader will not be distracted by the answers before reading the text. The disease entity listed is the correct diagnosis for each of the 27 cases presented. A detailed index including *all* gastrointestinal disorders considered in the text is also provided for easy reference.

Index

NOTE: The entries in **bold type** indicate the gastrointestinal disorders discussed in detail in the text and the page references.

NOTE: The entries in **bold type** indicate the
gastrointestinal disorders discussed in detail in the text and the page references.

Cholangiography
for differential diagnosis of pancreatitis
and cholecystitis, 196
value of tomography, 193, 196
Cholecystectomy, 193
Cholecystitis
acute, dilatation of transverse colon and,
76
and gallstones, 197
associated with cystic duct obstruction,
196
emphysematous, 70–74
bacteria in gallbladder, 74
diabetes mellitus and, 74
diagnostic signs, 73
gallstones and, 71, 74
incidence of, 74
obstruction of cystic duct, 74
Cholecystitis glandularis proliferans, 194
Cholecystography
Cholografin, 196
Telepaque, 193, 196
Cholografin, characteristics of, 196
Cholecystography, visualization of adenomyoma, 194–195
Cirrhosis, hepatic varices, 22–23
Colitis
amebic, 5, 10—11, 13
differential diagnosis of ulcerative and
granulomatous colitis, 180–182
**granulomatous, 3, 8–9, 12, 13–16, 147,
169, 171, 174–177, 180–182**
"cobblestones," 146, 179
"collar button" ulcers, 177, 180
diarrhea and, 174, 176
differentiation of "pseudopolyps" from
true polyps, 179
excentric involvement, 8
fissure-like ulcers, 177, 182
fistula formation, 3, 12
hemorrhage in, 12
infrequent involvement of rectum, 171
involvement of terminal ileum, 9, 171,
180
limitation to right colon, 171
mimicking ileocecal tuberculosis, 143–
146
obstruction in, 12
pseudopolyps, 43, 45, 146, 171, 179
"skin lesions," 8, 12–14, 171, 177

NOTE: The entries in **bold type** indicate the
gastrointestinal disorders discussed in detail in the text and the page references.

"skip lesions", 5, 12, 14
"string sign", 12
mucus, erroneous diagnosis of, 89
ulcerative, 2–16, 169, 171, 177, 220
bloody stools and, 12
carcinoma of colon and. 12
circumferential involvement, 5, 13, 14
"collar button" appearance, 5, 9, 12–14,
177, 180, 182
continuity of involvement 5, 13
hemorrhage in, 12
improbability of mimicking ileocecal
tuberculosis, 146–147
left colon involvement, 180
perforation and, 12
pseudopolyps, 171
"spiculated" appearance, 5, 9, 13
toxic megacolon and, 12, 76, 181
Colitis cystica profunda, characteristics, 43,
45, 169
Colon
abnormal position of in midgut volvulus,
96, 97, 100, 269
cathartic, 5, 11–13
chronic use of laxatives, 11–12
diverticulum of, 76
endometriosis of, 240–241
symptoms, 241
hamartoma of, 241
leiomyoma of, 240
lipoma of, 238–244
lymphosarcoma of, 141–142, 147, 166–
169
microcolon, 161
perforated, and necrotizing enterocolitis,
156
scleroderma of, **179–180**
sigmoid
"coffee bean" sign of volvulus, 105, 112
lymphoma of, 172
toxic megacolon, 12, 76, 181
transverse
dilatation of, 73, 76
lymphoma of, 172
ulcers, 5, 9–11, 13–14
vascular occlusion of (see Vascular occlusion, of colon)
Constipation, pneumatosis cystoides intestinalis and, 42
Crohn's disease
diagnostic signs, 55, **58**–59, 171, 220
"creeping fat," 117, 121
differentiation from Whipple's disease,
120

NOTE: The entries in **bold type** indicate the gastrointestinal disorders discussed in detail in the text and the page references.

NOTE: The entries in **bold type** indicate the gastrointestinal disorders discussed in detail in the text and the page references.

NOTE: The entries in **bold type** indicate the gastrointestinal disorders discussed in detail in the text and the page references.

NOTE: The entries in **bold type** indicate the
gastrointestinal disorders discussed in detail in the text and the page references.

NOTE: The entries in **bold type** indicate the gastrointestinal disorders discussed in detail in the text and the page references.

NOTE: The entries in **bold type** indicate the gastrointestinal disorders discussed in detail in the text and the page references.

NOTE: The entries in **bold type** indicate the
gastrointestinal disorders discussed in detail in the text and the page references.

NOTE: The entries in **bold type** indicate the gastrointestinal disorders discussed in detail in the text and the page references.